MUM,
CAN I EAT THIS?

A collection of my recipes to share with
anyone who requires low fructose,
low FODMAP, table-sugar free, gluten free,
and low or no lactose foods

CASEY ELLIS

Editor: Claire McGregor
Project management and text design: Michael Hanrahan Publishing
Cover design: Peter Reardon
Photographer: Julie Renouf
Food stylist: Cherise Pagano
Food preparation: Casey Ellis

DISCLAIMER & IMPORTANT NOTICE

The author and publisher of this cook book is not a dietitian, doctor or healthcare professional. The ingredients listed for the recipes have been checked and confirmed by Janelle Couch, Accredited Practising Dietitian as being appropriate for anyone requiring recipes that contain ingredients that are low FODMAP* and free of gluten and sucrose (table sugar). Although the ingredients have been checked by an Accredited Practising Dietitian, some of the ingredients may not be appropriate or suitable for your specific medical condition or dietary requirements. Before using a recipe you should check the ingredients to ensure that they are appropriate and suitable for your specific medical condition or dietary requirements. You should always consult your doctor or dietitian and obtain professional medical advice before commencing any modified diet.

_____

* FODMAP is an acronym for **F**ermentable **O**ligosaccharides **D**isaccharides **M**onosaccharides **A**nd **P**olyols.

Contents

Introduction **1**
Our story **3**
Hints and tips **13**
Master ingredients list **15**

Savoury

Beef stock **18**
Chicken stock **20**
Cucumber and cherry tomato salad **21**
Crusty crumbed chicken legs **22**
Beef tacos **24**
Chicken noodle soup **26**
Chicken soup **28**
Cottage pie **30**
Egg and chive pasta with lamb
   cutlets **32**
Fettucine carbonara **34**
Homemade hamburgers **36**
Lamb stew **38**
Lasagne **40**
Mini pizzas **42**
Moussaka **44**
Oven spaghetti **46**
Peri peri chicken **48**
Pumpkin soup **50**
Red chicken **52**
Red spaghetti and meatballs **54**

Rice paper rolls **56**
Roast lamb, veggies and gravy **58**
Savoury rice **60**
Spaghetti Bolognese **62**
Stuffed capsicums **64**
Meatballs and salsa dip **66**
Tomato salsa **67**
Meat sauce and rice **70**
Tomato, cheese and chive muffins **72**
Tuna mornay **74**
Tuna salad **76**

Sweet

Anzac biscuits **80**
Chocolate biscuits **81**
Gingernut biscuits **82**
Shortbread biscuits **84**
Vanilla biscuits **85**
Baked custard **86**
Banana and blueberry cake **88**
Banana milkshake **90**
Caramel milkshake **91**
Chocolate milkshake **92**
Strawberry milkshake **93**
Caramel sundae **96**
Chocolate sundae **97**
Banana split **98**

Blueberry crumble **100**

Custard **102**

Blueberry jam **103**

Raspberry jam **104**

Strawberry jam **106**

Caramel sauce **107**

Chocolate sauce **108**

Chocolate brownies **110**

Chocolate cupcakes **112**

Vanilla cupcakes **113**

Vanilla and blueberry cupcakes **116**

Banana ice-cream **117**

Chocolate ice-cream **118**

Passionfruit ice-cream **119**

Vanilla ice-cream **120**

Fruit and marshmallow skewers **122**

Chocolate mousse **124**

Lemon slice **126**

Marshmallows **128**

Peanut brittle **129**

Toffees **130**

Mixed berry and banana sorbet **132**

Blueberry cheesecake **134**

Raspberry cheesecake **135**

Strawberry cheesecake **138**

Orange fizzy drink **139**

Orange and lemon fizzy drink **140**

Pancakes **142**

Pavlova with passionfruit cream **144**

Rumballs **146**

Scones with strawberry jam and cream **148**

Vanilla and chocolate marble cake **150**

Sweetened condensed milk **152**

Whipped cream **153**

Cook's notes **154**

Meal plans **154**

Index **155**

Acknowledgements **156**

Introduction

When life gives you lemons, make lemonade, right? Well, what if you have an intolerance and can't have lemonade? Or, worse yet, your child does? When you are forced to watch your child go through the pain and suffering that comes with intolerances, it rips your heart out.

To ease that pain and suffering in our family, and to add a little normality and joy, I took to the stove. After all, it's hard enough being a kid these days without missing out on the things you love and being distinguished as 'different'. After much trial and error, I have created a degree of normality in my children's lives, and it tastes amazing!

I am not a dietitian, doctor or health care professional. I am a Mum, who wanted to share some recipes that work for my children. I have published this collection to share with everyone suffering from fructose, gluten, sucrose (sugar), IBS and lactose intolerances, but most of all for the kids. I would add, though, that if you or your child regularly suffer from abdominal discomfort, see a Medical Specialist. You may assume you have fructose or lactose intolerance, for example, but only a Medical Specialist can diagnose this and rule out anything more serious. Although the wait might be long, have courage and don't give up! The ingredients list has been approved by an Accredited Practising Dietitian. Please get the Master Ingredients list approved by your health care professional to ensure it is suitable for you.

Several years ago, my daughter Keira and, later, her sister Madison were diagnosed with intolerances. It was so overwhelming. There was a lack of credible information and certainly a lack of cookbooks that catered for children. Sure, there were a few low FODMAP books out there, but certainly nothing that was catering for children. Most of the recipes I did find, my daughter would never eat, and as for fun food that you would find at a party – so that she could feel like everyone else – well, these recipes were even scarcer, and usually had that not-quite-right, earthy taste that we refer to in our house as a 'hippie food taste'. Keira wanted things to taste like the food she'd had before she was diagnosed.

Then when it came time to teach my husband how to cook for her, well, there was no way he could do so. If it isn't written down exactly, then forget it. That is when it began, this idea for a cookbook as a way to help other parents, carers and friends. A way to make everything just that bit easier for the children; they were my inspiration. So here is our story.

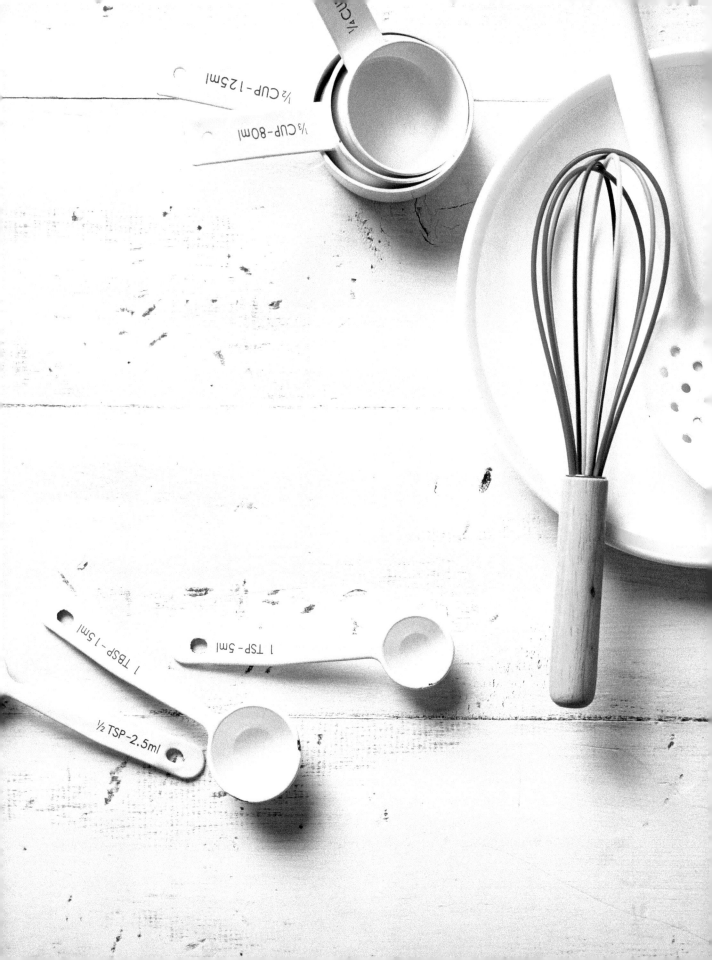

Our story

My daughter Keira had always just been one of those happy-go-lucky children. You know the ones who find it easy to make friends, enjoys school and whom every teacher likes? Then, one non-specific day, at age five, she came down with gastro. It completely wrecked her, but true to her personality she was stoic. She required a bucket so often we covered one with glittery stickers. Forty-eight hours later she couldn't sleep without being sick on herself, and so we went to ED, where she was given a nausea suppressant.

When she got better we thought nothing more about it. Little did we know that this episode may have been the catalyst for the most challenging, emotional and physically taxing time of our lives to date.

Over the next few months, Keira would sporadically complain of feeling unwell. As she was young, I thought nothing much about it; just kiddie bugs, surely? I would just check her when she said this, and she would lay on the couch or even miss school occasionally, much to her dismay.

Now, stomach issues run in my family, and so I have had a lot of experience with doctors, and this led to my mind beginning to tick over. I decided to take Keira to the doctors as I had noticed that she had distention (bloating) of her abdomen. I knew from experience that this could be a sign of faecal loading (constipation), and that this can make you feel ill.

The first doctor we saw felt her abdomen and told me she was indeed faecally loaded, and that she should take some laxatives to 'clear her out', and he sent me on my way. This seemed reasonable to me and so I followed the instructions, but after a week it seemed that the problem had not resolved and Keira was still complaining. In fact, it seemed to be getting worse; she lost the colour in her face, sometimes for the better part of the day, as well as feeling constantly nauseated. I resolved to get this fixed and this time went to see another helpful GP. He sent Keira for x-rays, which showed that she did indeed have considerable faecal loading. This was it – I decided I needed to act.

The doctor again wanted to prescribe laxatives; I politely asked to be referred to a specialist instead, which he kindly did. I rang to make an appointment but we couldn't get in to see him for a month! I could not wait that long – my daughter was ill. Keira had now progressed to feeling ill daily. She was constantly pale, had stomach cramps, was lethargic and nauseated. Occasionally, she would get diarrhoea and sit on the toilet with a bucket, while shaking and dry retching or vomiting. It was heartbreaking.

At this time, I was studying part-time at uni, but this was becoming untenable. I had reduced to just one unit and managed a pass mark, but the pressure was building. In the end I just could not keep up. I was severely sleep-deprived (Keira would wake at all hours, usually one or two o'clock in the morning) and I had little study time. I then failed by the barest of margins and subsequently failed my first subject ever. At that moment I knew the only thing I could do was to defer. It was another trial in an increasingly difficult path.

Waiting one month to see the specialist was too long. I explained the situation to the receptionist but to no avail. I then asked if the specialist practised at any other location, which he did. I called there and was elated to get an earlier appointment, I also left my daughter's name at both locations on the cancellation list. Thankfully, we saw the specialist just one week later.

The specialist was lovely with Keira and asked her a number of questions, mostly about school. I realised then what he was getting at as he moved on to me. 'Does she enjoy school? Does she have a lot of friends?' I knew what he was doing and it irritated me because if I had thought for one second that this had anything to do with a psychological cause, I would have gone straight to a psychologist! I knew then that we were going to butt heads, but I was here for my daughter and so I tried to keep calm.

'No!' I replied. 'She loves school, is a very good student, has a lot of friends who we have over for play dates, and she misses them as she is missing a tremendous amount of school.'

'Why is she missing school?'

'Well, let me see…' and I explained the situation.

'Yes, well, she is only constipated!'

I could have kicked him in the shins! I explained, as calmly as I could, how she is very clearly sick, how she complains of feeling sick and that she has no colour in her face. I said that anyone can see she is sick. I also explained how occasionally I had sent her to school only for them to send her home again. Keira goes to a public school and it is not their responsibility to look after a sick child – they have enough to do without that too.

Finally, he examined my daughter and prescribed OsmoLax, in a high dosage, to clear her out. I questioned why this had happened to Keira and if there could be an underlying problem. He said that he felt that it was simply a case of severe constipation, and that Keira would be better in seven days.

Personally, I am all about facts and plausibility, and this scenario seemed plausible; after all, he was the expert. I took him at his word and left with hopes high. But one week later I emailed him to say there was no change with Keira. In fact, she seemed worse. She was now not sleeping well and we were waking at all hours with her on the toilet. She cried most days and my heart was breaking; I was becoming desperate.

The specialist replied that we should wait a week or two for her stomach to settle down and all would be well. In the meantime, I visited my father to talk it over with him. My father has always been my sounding board. He, too, agreed that there was something not right. Once the faecal loading had gone, she should have begun to feel better. Something else was going on, but what?

Trust your gut

I started to spend my now-sleepless nights trawling the internet, typing in her symptoms and looking at medical articles, blogs and websites. I read about intolerances to fructose and lactose where the symptoms sounded like Keira's. The problem was that the symptoms also said 'diarrhoea', whereas Keira only had diarrhoea when the constipation became too much; called faecal overloading. I knew I needed to talk this over with Keira's GP.

I know a lot of doctors like a person's symptoms to fit into 'the box' – that the clinically observed list of symptoms point to one specific ailment. I researched many, many blogs and chat boards and poured over different people's experiences, and found that many others were exhibiting similar symptoms to Keira's: constipation, nausea and lethargy; these were the main culprits.

I kept coming across the same things and so I just knew that I needed to get her the appropriate tests. A hydrogen test seemed the easiest and least painful way to confirm what I suspected – that she was fructose or lactose intolerant. I didn't know which it would be, or both.

I wrote again to her specialist and told him of all that had been going on. I told him of all the crying too. I said that I thought it might be an intolerance, specifically to fructose. I received an email reply and he said that he did not agree, as the pattern was not typical for a carbohydrate intolerance (fructose/lactose) but that he would be happy to see us again. I could have cried but, as always, I had to be mindful that my daughter was in close proximity.

A few nights before, at about 2 am, when Keira was shaking, pale, nauseated and sitting on the toilet crying, I had held her head between my hands and looked her in the eyes and promised her I would get her better. No matter how many doctors it took, I would find a way. I took a deep breath and made another appointment with a fantastic GP that had become Keira's GP. I had found him the most helpful and hopeful so far, not for saying, 'I know what is wrong with Keira,' but for saying, 'I have done all I can, and I still don't know, but I will help you find out. I will send you to whomever we need to, to get to the bottom of this.' I will forever be grateful for his truthfulness and support.

I made an appointment with him and we discussed the problem again. I told him my theory and he thought it was plausible, although he explained why my fructose theory was more likely than lactose. He said that lactose intolerance is something you are more likely to be born with, though not always. I felt empowered from the visit. Next, I made an appointment with a lovely local dietitian to run the idea by her. We spoke about Keira's symptoms and she too thought the fructose intolerance was plausible. She gave me a list of low-FODMAP ingredients as a start and said that I should notice an improvement in three to four weeks.

I came away and realised that the list was quite restrictive. *What am I going to feed Keira?* I thought. *What can I cook? She won't eat this stuff; she is going to starve!* Anxiety began to fill me anew. To add to this, I found that any cookbooks that catered for these FODMAP's or were low fructose, our children did not find overly exciting. Well, as expected, Keira hated the food! After a few days, and a lot of complaining, we decided that as it was Easter the following week, and we didn't want to put her through this if we were wrong, we would wait for a diagnosis before starting any special diets.

Easter came and Keira got another bout of gastro. When she had recovered she started to run around and play like she was well again. She even said to her dad and I with enthusiasm, 'I'm fixed!' But she was sick again a couple of days later. I now know it would have been because her system had been 'cleaned out'.

An uphill struggle

I headed to the next specialist appointment, which was three days later. The room was tense as the specialist again started asking Keira about school. I stopped him and told him the story of a friend I knew. I told him how the doctors tried to pigeonhole her and say it was all psychological because they couldn't come up with a plausible diagnosis. I told him that it turned out she really did have a physiological issue and not a psychological one. I said that he would not be doing that to my child. He was clearly not happy with what I had said. I told him that I wanted the hydrogen tests. He replied that he thought it was unwarranted, but that he would do them because, he said, 'I wouldn't want you to say, "I told you so!"'

His solution instead was to recommend putting my now six-year-old daughter under anaesthesia for a gastroscopy. He said that in the absence of any other plausible diagnosis, this was the next option as, so far, her blood test results and faecal testing had come back as normal. I knew that he was not taking this decision lightly. I took a deep breath and asked about the risks and what it would entail. I asked him, 'What choice do I have?' He told me it was up to me.

I knew that it was at least plausible that I was right, but, if I was wrong, it was more time my daughter had to wait, and she was sick. I left in a quandary but when I got to my car I immediately made the appointment for the hydrogen tests the specialist had consented to. There was a three-month wait. I pleaded with the receptionist and she said she could fit us in in a month, but that there may not be a seat for us as we were being squeezed in. I told her I would sit on the floor if necessary, and Keira could sit on my knee.

A couple of days later we were back with our local GP. I was beginning to feel like we were always there, and that Keira was becoming too familiar with the inside of doctors' offices. This time, she was doubled over in pain and was crying. Although he was patient and kind, as usual, there was nothing he could do. I told him about the specialist appointment and asked him if it was his daughter, what would he do? He told me the same thing I had already concluded myself: she has to have the gastroscopy. I decided that if I was wrong about the fructose and lactose, it was time lost, and a gastroscopy was an opportunity to find the real problem.

We had started to take sick bags everywhere we went now; Keira had gotten worse. She was regularly dry retching, no matter where we were. Also in my bag of tricks was toilet paper. Keira hated the toilet paper in the doctors' offices, so the only solution was for me to carry our own. I remember the looks I got when I pulled it out of my bag, which ranged from curious to downright disgusted.

I had a mountain of doctors' certificates for Keira's school, and she had missed about three months of school by that stage. I always tried to keep them updated and went in regularly to pick up work for her. I began to worry that what I was teaching Keira was not catering to what she needed in terms of schooling, so I resolved to talk about home schooling with our lovely GP the next time I saw him.

A worrying time

The day of the gastroscopy arrived and I still hadn't told Keira what was going on. I was hoping not to alarm her; she hated the blood tests she had already had, and I knew she would ask me if she had to have a needle. We arrived early. My husband dropped us off as he had to work, and my mum was looking after my youngest. After waiting for a little while, I began to tell Keira what was going to happen. I said they were going to put her to sleep and she asked why. I told her that they wanted to have a look inside her tummy and that the only way to do that was to put a camera in there. I told her that maybe we could get pictures – how awesome! She was scared. I told her to try not to be, that I would be with her when she went to sleep and when she woke up. She cried a little and I just hugged her. I was trying to be strong but inside I was nervous and a little scared too.

A nurse came in and we went through the pre-op questions. The nurses were amazing – so caring. They explained that they were giving her some numbing cream for her hand so that it wouldn't hurt when they gave her the needle. The specialist came in and I thought to myself that at least he is always lovely with Keira. I held her hand and stayed with her until she was asleep.

My wait in the waiting room was horrible. Not only was I worrying for my daughter but I was hearing the stories from the other mothers around me of their children. Children who were born with poorly formed oesophagi and who couldn't eat properly and needed regular operations. I knew that things could have been a lot worse, I did know that, but everyone's situation is relative. All I knew was that my child couldn't function; she was always pale, tired, nauseated, dry retching or spending hours on the toilet. We, too, needed a solution.

After about an hour, the specialist came out and told me that all had gone well and that Keira would be waking up soon. He said they had found *nothing abnormal.* I breathed a sigh of relief and groaned internally; it had all been for nothing.

I was called in to her bedside when she was starting to stir. I was sitting with her when she woke up; her eyes were huge. She kept opening and closing her mouth. Her lips were a little puffy from the tubes and she had red marks for the tape. 'Mummy,' she whispered. I hugged her and, seeing her like that, I wanted to cry. I had put her through this for nothing. What if something had happened to her? It would have been my fault.

Apart from her gastrointestinal problems, Keira was always getting sick. If there was a virus, cold or flu within a 500-metre radius, she would catch it. In order to get a hydrogen test, you need to have not taken antibiotics in the two weeks prior to the test. One week before the appointment, the one we had been waiting a month for, Keira got sick and needed antibiotics. Argh! I rang to cancel and reschedule the test. It was the same woman and we had the same conversation. Again, we would have to wait another month and again we were to sit on the floor.

'I told you so!'

Many GP visits and more sleepless nights later, the day had come. The first test was a lactulose test used as a baseline. On that day we sat on the floor for three hours and met some amazing people, one of whom was a primary school teacher. I explained my schooling issues to her and she kindly gave me some fabulous advice about apps for Keira for both English and Math. She showed me the benchmarks that Keira should be meeting. Over the three days we were there she helped to teach me how to teach Keira. I can't tell you how grateful I am to her for her kindness.

The lactose test was on the second day, and this was negative. Finally, on the third day, we came to the fructose test. I was so nervous. What would I do if this came back negative too? Keira drank her cup of solution and then the nurse went through the instructions. Over what was supposed to be a three-hour test, Keira would blow into a machine every 15 minutes. This was the same process as the previous two tests, and then we waited for the results. You know you have tested positive if you go above a certain reading a couple of times. It took just one hour to ascertain that Keira was fructose intolerant; her readings were through the roof.

I was elated and overwhelmed all at once. I was handed a brochure about what Keira should and shouldn't eat. I was told to make an appointment with her specialist for the following week. As opposed to the other times, I made this appointment almost gleefully. After months of struggle and having to push the agenda, I would finally get to see him and not have him look at my daughter with disbelieving eyes.

My husband and family were elated that finally we could help Keira. They had all been putting on a brave face, but I knew they were worried. My husband was having to work through it all, as well as my parents, whose support had been invaluable. Thinking back, I remember one night several months into Keira being ill when my daughters wanted to stay at Nan and Pop's. They were so excited that I didn't have the heart to say no, but I was worried. I told my parents to call if there was a problem, to which they replied, 'We raised five children – there is nothing we can't handle.'

I received a call at about 11.30 pm that night; they didn't know what to do. Keira was doubled over on the toilet and they were telling her she needed to go home. She was getting upset as she didn't want to go. She was shaking and sweating so I went around to pick her up. They wanted me to take her to the ED. I said, 'Why? What will they do? They don't know how to help; they don't know what's wrong.'

During that whole conversation, all I could think was *welcome to my life*. I picked her up and took her home with tears in my eyes.

But nights like that were going to be all over now – now I could finally fix my little girl.

When I arrived at the appointment with Keira's specialist, he seemed aloof. Looking at her file he said, 'Oh, yes, I see that she has a fructose intolerance, well…' Then nothing. I felt the response was insufficient.

I asked the questions I had: How did she acquire this? Is it hereditary? Will it go away? etc. He answered with little emotion and I resolved to change doctors after the visit. I left thinking to myself that if I had not pushed the point, if I had not done the research and believed in my daughter when it felt as though almost no one else did, if I did not have the strength of character to do so, to advocate for her, she would still be sick. How was that fair?

There are many people out there who do not know what questions to ask or what specialist to be sent to. If in doubt ask, and always trust your gut. I think the medical profession does a truly amazing job, and for that I respect them. That does not mean, however, that there should not be give and take. Everyone should be able to walk away with the same positive outcome for their child as I did with mine. You are your child's best advocate.

The way forward

My next task was possibly just as scary – walking into a supermarket. Did you know that almost everything in a supermarket has fructose in it? Well it does. After crying in the supermarket aisle and having people look at me strangely, I left and ended up finding an amazing paediatric dietitian. She gave me a detailed list of the things Keira could and couldn't have, a few recipes that my daughter said tasted like dirt, and then left me to my own devices.

Armed with the comprehensive information, I was well on my way and we began. After about three weeks, Keira was able to get up off the couch. I remember the day she began to smile again. The bad news was that she hated almost everything I fed her. I bought low FODMAP books and looked at low-fructose books, too, but most of the recipes she hated. I would say they had a 'hippie flavour'; sort of earthy and bitter with an odd aftertaste. So, I started a test kitchen where I would take a recipe and tweak it over and over until it tasted like something she would have eaten prior to her intolerance diagnosis.

I have been doing this for several years now, using my husband, his boss and work colleagues as guinea pigs too. I have come up with some pretty easy and quick low-fructose and no-sucrose recipes (oh yeah, she has that problem too: Keira has problems tolerating foods with excess anything with fructans, GOS, polyols, fructose or sucrose (sugar).) I make the recipes for friends – anyone really – and nobody generally knows the difference between a cake I would have cooked before to now.

After Keira was diagnosed and we adjusted her diet, her health greatly improved, and she was able to return to school on a more regular basis. We still have plenty of medical appointments but, for the majority of the time, Keira is attending school regularly. With the help of a tutor she is catching up and is now enjoying school again. I, too, was able to get back to studying and I am currently in my final year of university.

When I first found out about Keira's intolerances I was so overwhelmed and often thought how amazing it would be to have a children's recipe book with recipes a child would actually eat. A recipe book that would allow your child to feel included so that they, too, could have the fun foods that their friends had. Whether at school, a friend's, or hosting a party – they wouldn't have to miss out. A book that could save another's heartache and headache because they knew what to cook. So, here it is! I hope it helps. This is my labour of love and ode to my daughters, Keira and Madison.

Hints and tips

Birthday parties. How heartbreaking is it when you have to watch your child miss out at a birthday party? When you have to look into their face and see the jealousy, disappointment, longing and in the beginning or on a bad day, the tears that fall. I've lost track of the amount of times I witnessed this, particularly in those early years when I was fine-tuning and BINNING my creations. Now, we simply call ahead to the person hosting the party and get a list of foods that will be there. I then delve into my repertoire of recipes and match the food as closely as possible. This saves me having to explain things to the host, makes me feel more comfortable and, ultimately and most importantly, allows my child to truly participate in the fun of a birthday party. Bye, bye tears.

Heading out for dinner? A little preparation will save you a lot of embarrassment. First things first, work out where you want to go and download the menu. Work out what you can eat. Are there any changes that need to be made to a particular dish? Ring the restaurant ahead of time and ask any questions you may have, such as: 'Do you pre-make your salads?', 'Can you take out the onion?', or 'Are your chips beer-battered?' and 'What do you put in your mashed potatoes?'

When you are ordering, always make sure that they know it's for a customer with an intolerance. A lot of restaurants are reluctant to accommodate people who they believe are on fad diets or just don't like things. When you take the time to explain it is for an intolerance and that the food will make your child sick, you will be amazed at what can be done. Always ensure that if there is a language barrier you seek out someone who understands completely. I learnt that lesson the hard way and it's always your child who pays the price!

Every child with fructose is different. What one child can tolerate is not necessarily what another one can. I recommend seeing a specialist for diagnosis and a paediatric dietitian to help you get started, but make sure it is someone who specialises in intolerances. When we finally found our paediatric dietitian she was worth her weight in gold.

The changes are sort of working. Just because your child has been diagnosed with fructose intolerance/malabsorption, for example, doesn't mean that there isn't something else going on. When Keira was diagnosed she was 100% better a few weeks after we changed her diet. However, over time, she would still have intermittent bouts of nausea and/or diarrhoea. It turns out she has problems with more than just fructose. It was combined with some bowel issues, so you can see how this might cause some issues. The bottom line is, if things aren't right, there may be other issues, so explore these with your specialist or paediatric dietitian. Remember: You are the best advocate for your child – trust your gut.

Always read the labels. There are always hidden nasties in food that you never would have thought about. I always believed that my family had a well-balanced diet before Keira was diagnosed, and we did, mostly. Five food groups – tick. Beef casserole, anyone? Little things as simple as a beef stock cube can cause a heap of trouble for your child, so always make sure you read the labels. Onion powder, garlic powder, high-fructose corn syrup – these are staples in many pre-packaged foods.

Friends and family. Friends and family can be fantastic and supportive, but don't always know the consequences if they make a mistake when feeding your child. Don't be afraid to reiterate information to them whenever you feel it's necessary.

Where do I buy it? Now that you need to make almost everything from scratch, there are a few ingredients you will need to become familiar with, and also know where to buy them. Things such as dextrose powder, also known as glucose powder, you will be able to source from your local health food store. Xanthan gum and sugar-free pure vanilla extract can also be found at your local health food store or some major supermarkets. Rice malt syrup, gluten-free plain flour, gluten-free self-raising flour and gluten-free pasta can now be found at a cheaper price in the major supermarkets. If in doubt, ask your local health food store and they will generally be able to source what you need.

You can just change the recipe or create new ones. If you like a recipe in this book or any other book, don't be afraid to play around with the recipe and change it or create something completely new. Would that cake work with no dried fruit? Can I change the type of flour that is used? Will I need to adjust the cook time or oven temperature? If you can't tolerate sucrose (sugar), dextrose powder, or even rice malt syrup, look around at the available sweeters that you can tolerate, see what will work. Trial and error – that is all it takes. *Always consult your health care professional.* Make sure you make things fresh as you are not adding anything to preserve your food.

MASTER INGREDIENTS LIST

The ingredients list that inspired these recipes has been approved by an Accredited Practising Dietitian. Before using a recipe you should check the ingredients to ensure that they are appropriate and suitable for your specific medical condition or dietary requirements. Always eat in moderation. You should always consult your doctor or dietitian and obtain professional medical advice before commencing any modified diet.

Gluten-free self-raising flour
Gluten-free plain flour
Quinoa flakes
Gluten-free pasta
Rice
Pure cocoa powder
Gluten-free bicarb soda
Pure maple syrup
Coconut, shredded, dried
Gelatin
Allspice
Rosemary, fresh
Mint, fresh
Chilli flakes
Cinnamon, ground
Nutmeg, ground
Basil, fresh
Parsley, fresh
Vanilla extract pure, sugar free
Lactose-free cream cheese
Eggs
Lactose-free cheese
Parmesan cheese
Lactose-free sour cream
Oregano, dried
Butter
Lactose-free milk

Lactose-free thickened cream
Dextrose/glucose powder
Rice malt syrup
Rice wine vinegar
Xanthan gum
Paprika
Tomato paste
Tomato puree
Tomato, common
Tinned whole tomatoes
Cherry tomatoes
Potato
Parsnip
Carrot
Peanuts
Eggplant
Corn cob
Cucumber, common
Pumpkin, Jap
Chives
Spring onions (green tops only)
Capsicums
Ground ginger and fresh
Tuna
Oil
Peas, thawed
Water

Beef
Ham hock salt brined
Lamb
Chicken
Lemon
Orange
Blueberries
Strawberries
Raspberries
Banana (just ripened)
Passionfruit
Kiwi fruit
Pineapple
Gluten-free bread crumbs
Salt
Pepper
Gluten-free cornflour
Gluten-free rice noodles
Gluten-free rice paper rolls
Gluten-free yeast
Gluten-free hard taco shells
Gluten-free and low-FODMAP bread
Lettuce, Cos
Celery
Thyme, fresh
Sweet potato
Carbonated water

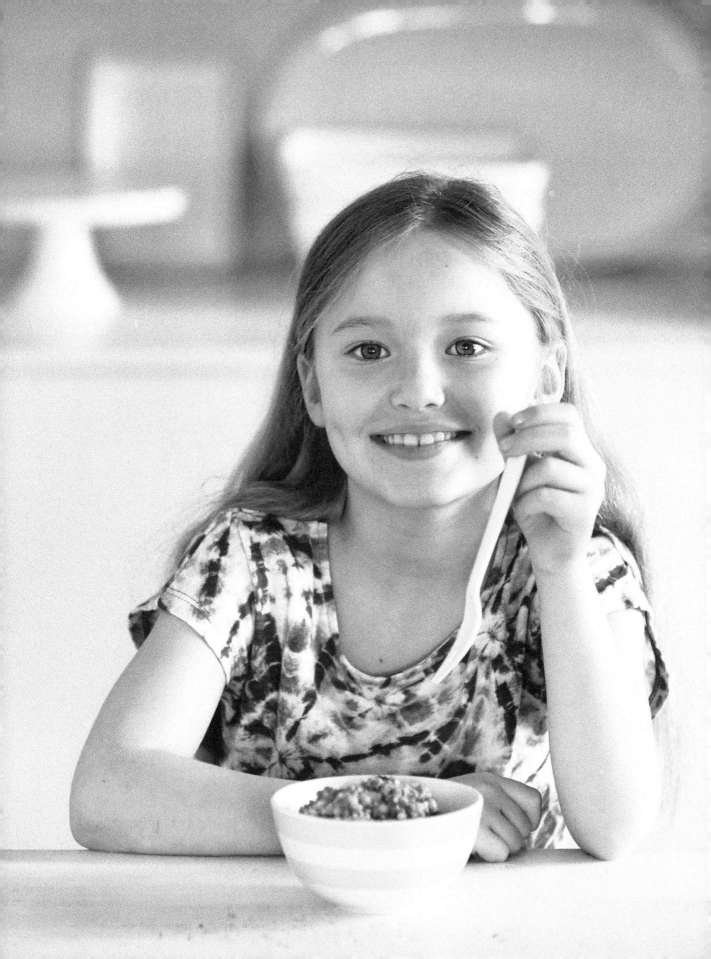

SAVOURY

Beef stock

Makes approx. 3 litres

1 tbsp olive oil

1 cup chives, roughly chopped

2½ kg beef bones

2 medium carrots, roughly chopped

½ cup parsley, roughly chopped

1½ tbsp salt

¼ tsp ground black pepper

2 sprigs thyme, fresh

4 litres water

Put the oil, chives, beef bones and carrots into a large stockpot. Fry until the bones have browned.

Add parsley, chives, salt, pepper, thyme and water. Bring to a boil then turn down to a simmer.

Simmer on low with lid on for 4 hours.

Season to taste

Pour stock through a fine sieve. Either use straight away or freeze.

Tip: Freeze in 1- or 2-cup batches in sandwich bags for ease of use in other recipes.

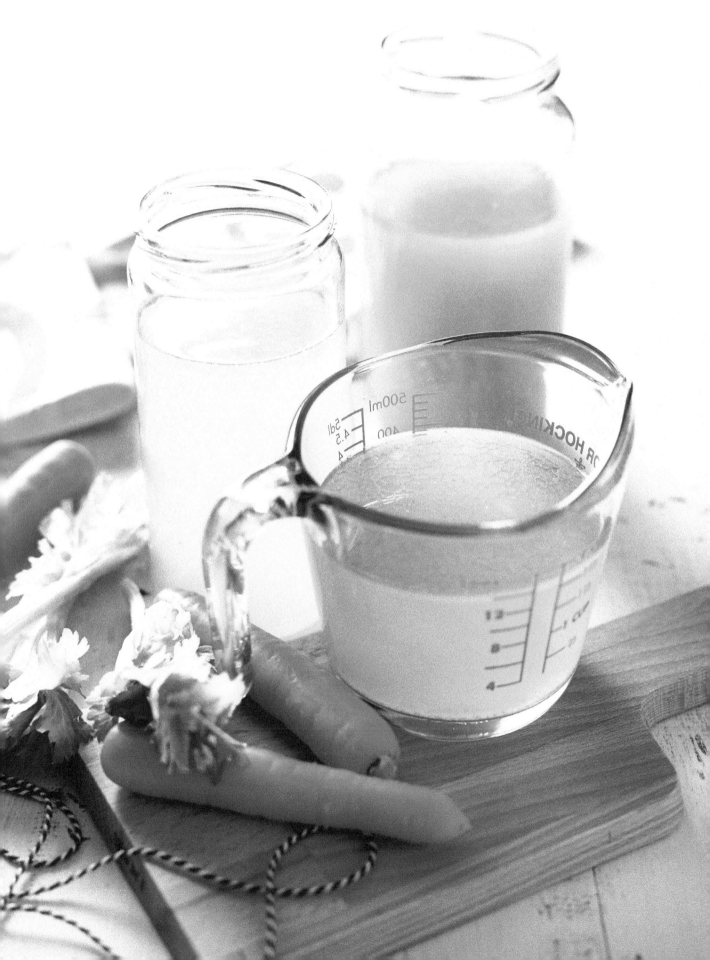

Chicken stock

Makes approx. 3 litres

1 tbsp olive oil

1 cup chives, roughly chopped

2½ kg chicken bones

¼ stick celery, roughly chopped

2 medium carrots, roughly chopped

⅓ cup parsley, roughly chopped

1½ tbsp salt

¼ tsp ground black pepper

4 litres water

Put the oil, chives, chicken bones, celery and carrots into a large stockpot. Fry until the bones have browned.

Add the parsley, salt, pepper and water. Bring to a boil then turn down to a simmer.

Simmer on low for 4 hours with the lid on.

Season to taste.

Pour stock through a fine sieve. Either use straight away or freeze.

Tip: Freeze in 1- or 2-cup batches in sandwich bags for ease of use in other recipes.

Cucumber and cherry tomato salad

Serves 4

250g punnet cherry tomatoes, halved

1 cucumber, common, diced

1 tbsp chives, finely chopped

½ tsp salt, extra to taste

20ml rice wine vinegar

35ml oil

Place tomatoes, cucumber, chives, salt, vinegar and oil in a salad bowl.

Toss well and add extra seasoning if required.

Serve.

Crusty crumbed chicken legs

Serves 4

500g chicken legs

Extra virgin olive oil

1 cup gluten-free dried breadcrumbs

⅛ tsp pepper

¼ tsp salt

Preheat oven to 180°C.

Place chicken legs in a large mixing bowl and coat liberally with oil.

Next, put the breadcrumbs, salt and pepper into a large sealable plastic bag.

Place the chicken legs into the plastic bag and coat well with the crumb mixture.

Place chicken legs onto an oven rack.

Cook for approx. 40–45 minutes, making sure to turn at least once, until golden brown and the juices run clear.

Serve.

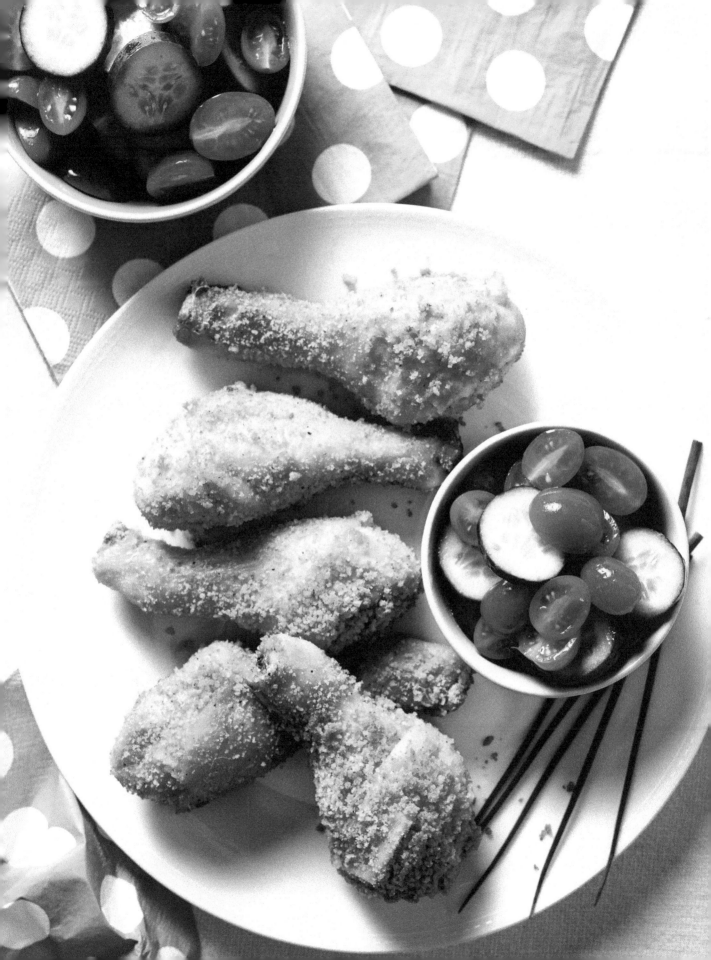

Beef tacos

Serves 4

Gluten-free hard taco shells

1 tsp olive oil

½ cup chives, chopped finely

500g beef mince

1 tsp salt

¾ tsp paprika

½ tsp dried chilli flakes

¼ cup water

¾ tsp oregano, dried

½ tbsp tomato paste

1 lettuce, cos

1 punnet cherry tomatoes, halved

1 cucumber, common, diced

Lactose-free sour cream (optional)

Salsa *(see recipe on page 67)*

250g lactose-free cheese, grated

Heat taco shells in oven according to instructions.

Into a medium saucepan over a medium heat, place the olive oil, chives and mince and cook until browned.

Add salt, paprika, dried chilli flakes, water, oregano and tomato paste. Combine well, cook for a further 5 minutes. Season to taste and then set aside.

Take a taco shell and fill with mince mixture, add a layer of lettuce, then tomato, cucumber, sour cream, salsa and finally the grated cheese.

Serve.

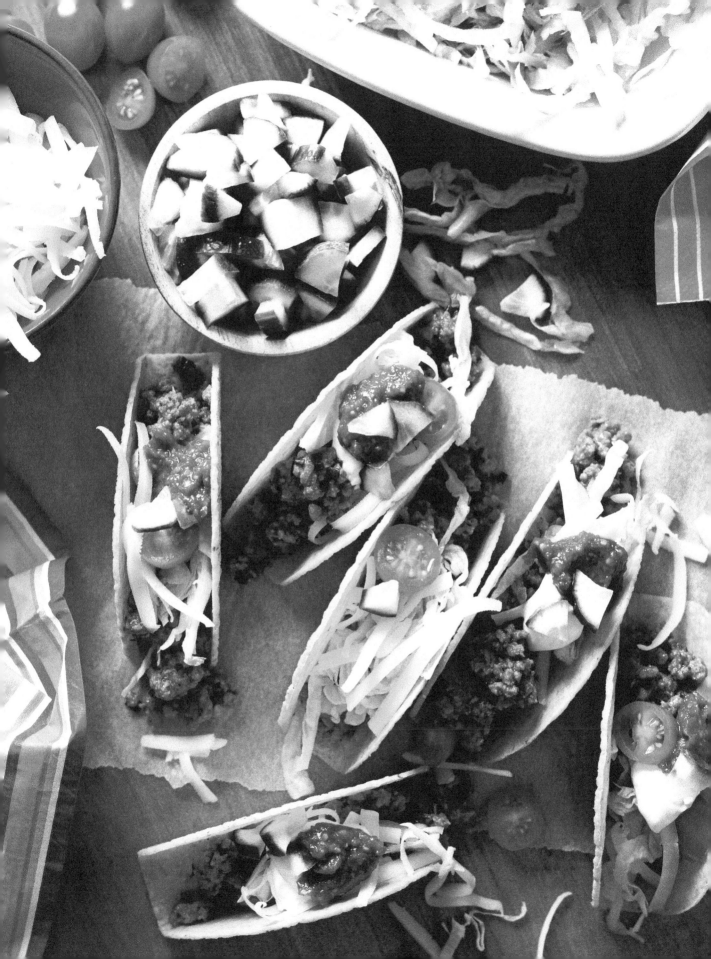

Chicken noodle soup

Serves 4

½ tbsp oil

300g chicken thigh fillets, thinly sliced

1 litre chicken stock *(see recipe on page 20)*

1 pack gluten-free rice noodles *(cook as per packet instructions)*

1 tbsp chives, finely chopped

Salt

Into a large saucepan over medium to high heat, place the oil and chicken. Cook chicken until browned.

Add chicken stock and allow to cook until chicken is well cooked (approx. 5 minutes).

Next, add the cooked rice noodles and chives and allow to simmer for a further minute.

Season to taste and serve.

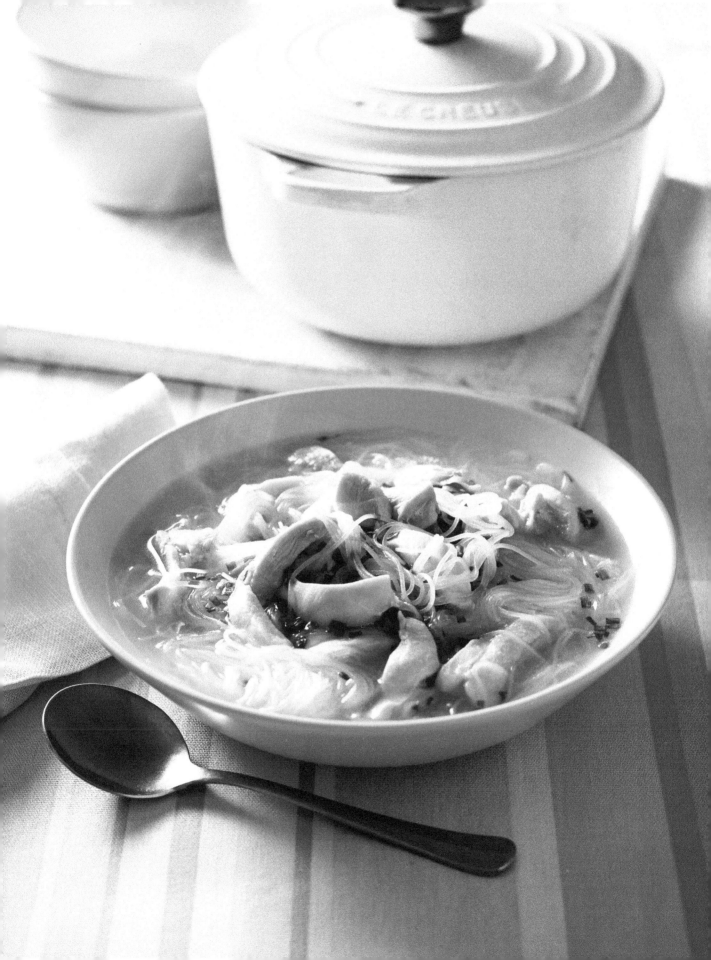

Chicken soup

Serves 6

1 tbsp olive oil

1.5kg chicken marylands

2 carrots, peeled, chopped

3 medium-sized potatoes, peeled, chopped into large cubes

¼ celery stick, diced

⅓ cup parsley, finely chopped

½ cup chives, finely chopped

1 parsnip, diced

Salt

Black pepper

2 litres chicken stock *(see recipe on page 20)*

½ cup water

Place oil and chicken in a large saucepan over a medium heat and fry until chicken is browned.

Add carrot, potatoes, celery, parsley, chives, parsnip as well as a seasoning of salt and pepper.

Pour in stock and water and bring to boil, then simmer for 1 hour and 30 minutes.

Take chicken out of pot and, using tongs, pull the chicken from the bones.

Discard bones and return the chicken meat to the pot.

Season to taste and serve.

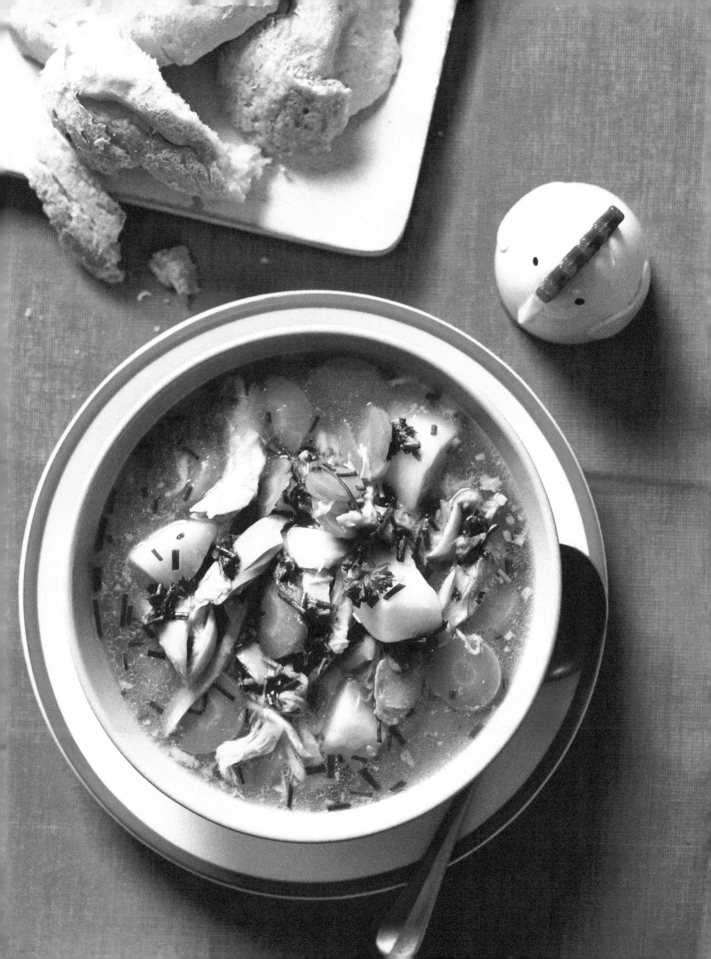

Cottage pie

Serves 6

1kg potatoes, diced

3 tbsp butter

½ cup lactose-free milk

1 tbsp oil

⅓ cup chives, chopped finely

500g beef mince

⅓ cup sweet potato, peeled and diced

1 carrot, chopped

¼ cup peas, thawed

½ cup diced pumpkin, Jap

2½ tsp oregano, dried

1 tsp salt

1 cup beef stock
(see recipe on page 18)

2½ tbsp dextrose powder

1 tin whole tomatoes

¼ cup tomato paste

100g lactose-free cheese, grated

Preheat oven to 180°C.

Place diced potatoes into a large saucepan of boiling water with a good pinch of salt and cook until soft.

Drain potatoes, place back into saucepan and mash with the butter and milk until well combined. Season to taste and set aside.

Place oil and chives in a medium saucepan over a medium heat and cook until chives have wilted. Add mince and cook until brown.

Next, add sweet potato, carrot, peas, pumpkin, oregano, salt, beef stock, dextrose powder, tomatoes and tomato paste.

Bring to boil and allow to simmer for 30 minutes or until vegetables are cooked.

Season to taste.

Place mince into the bottom of a 1.9 litre casserole dish and top with the mashed potato, and finally sprinkle with the cheese.

Place in oven for approx. 20 minutes or until golden brown.

Serve.

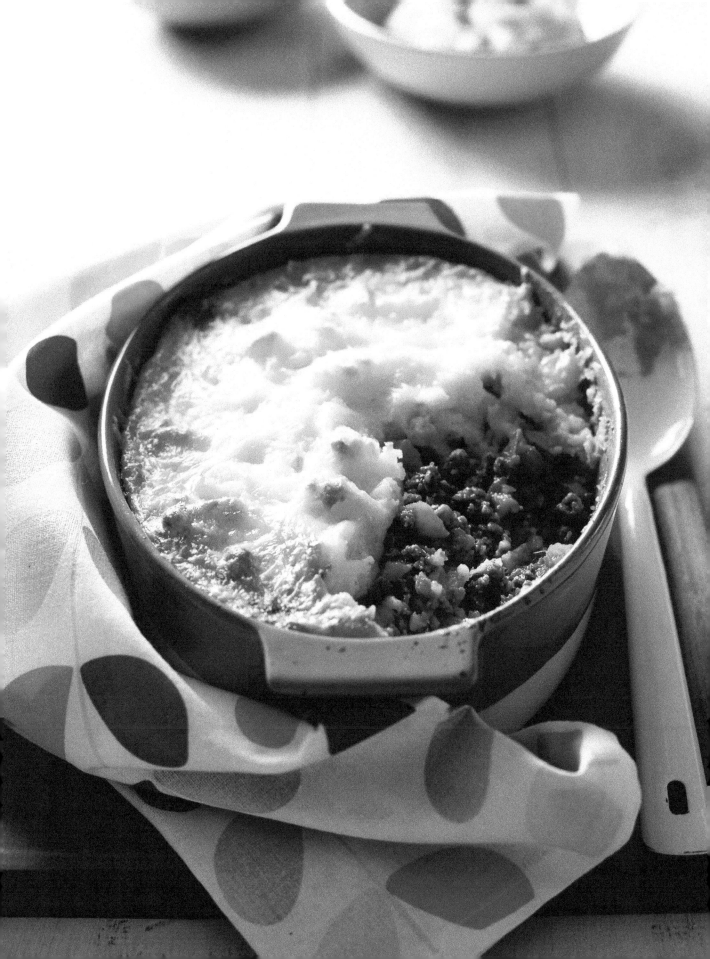

Egg and chive pasta with lamb cutlets

Serves 4

1 packet gluten-free pasta *(cooked as per packet instructions)*

8 lamb cutlets

1 tbsp oil

⅓ cup chives, finely chopped

4 eggs, beaten

½ tsp salt

Cook pasta and set aside.

Next, into a searing-hot large frying pan, place the seasoned, lamb cutlets and cook for approx. 2 minutes per side or until cooked to taste. Leave to rest.

Place oil and chives into a large saucepan and fry over medium heat for approx. 1 minute. Add the cooked pasta and combine well.

In a small bowl, beat eggs and add salt. Pour the egg mixture over the pasta and chive mixture and cook, stirring constantly, for approx. 1 minute or until egg has cooked.

Season to taste and serve.

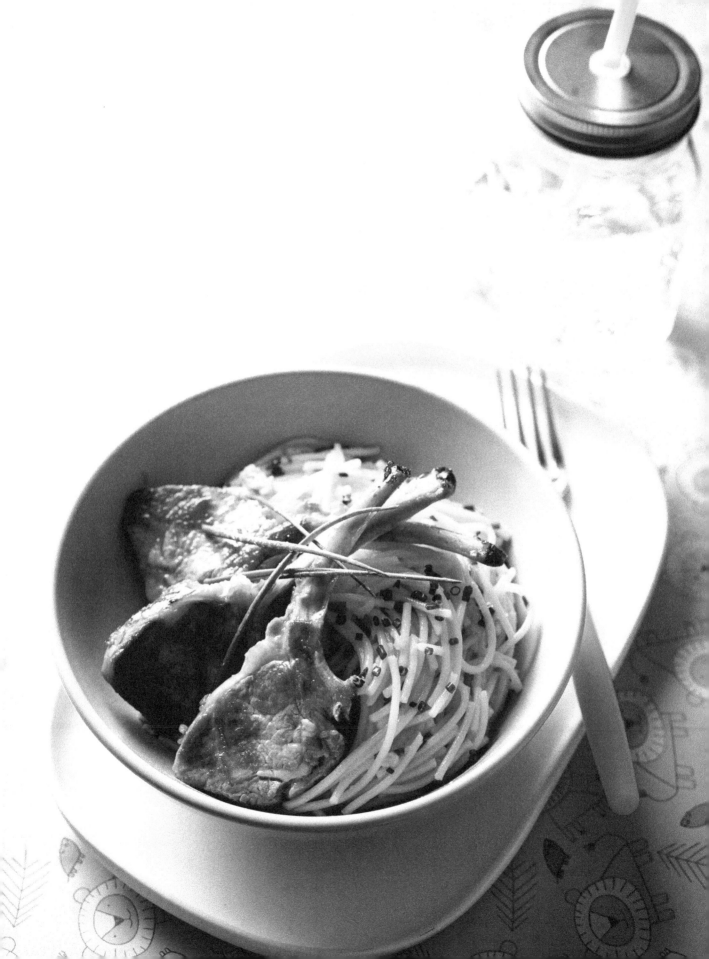

Fettucine carbonara

Serves 4

1 packet gluten-free fettucine

1 tbsp oil

1 cup ham hock salt brined; discard rind and finely dice

⅓ cup chives, finely chopped

⅔ cup lactose-free milk

1½ cups lactose-free cheese, grated

2 eggs, beaten

Salt

Pepper

Cook fettucine as per packet instructions.

Into a large saucepan, place the oil, ham hock and chives. Fry until it begins to brown.

Next, add ⅓ cup of the milk into the ham hock mixture and simmer for 1 minute.

In a separate medium mixing bowl, combine the cheese, eggs and remaining milk.

Add the fettucine and egg mixture to the ham hock mixture. Stir continuously over a very low heat until the cheese has melted.

Season to taste.

Serve.

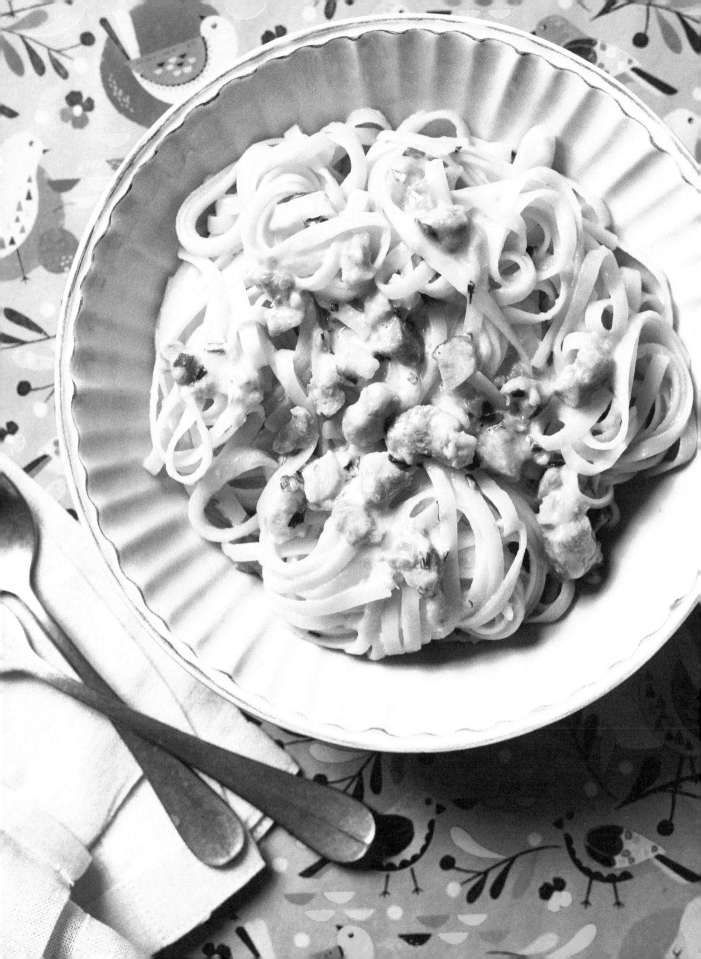

Homemade hamburgers

Serves 4

500g beef mince

¼ cup chives, finely chopped

5 eggs

½ tsp salt

2 tbsp gluten-free plain flour

2 tbsp olive oil

2 tomatoes, sliced

1 lettuce, cos

4 lactose-free cheese slices

8 pieces of gluten-free and low-FODMAP bread or 4 gluten-free and low-FODMAP bread rolls

Place mince, chives, 1 egg, salt and flour in a large mixing bowl. Use your hands to make sure the ingredients are incorporated well.

Roll the hamburger mixture into 4 balls.

Heat 1 tbsp of the oil in a large frying pan and then place the hamburgers into the pan. Using an egg flip, press the hamburger balls flat and allow each to brown on one side. Then flip over and brown on the other side. This will take approx. 3–4 minutes on each side.

Now, into another large frying pan, heat the remaining oil and fry the remaining 4 eggs, making sure to allow the eggs to have some movement in the middle.

To assemble the burgers, place a layer of tomato onto a slice of bread, then a layer of lettuce, a layer of cheese and finishing with the beef patty and fried egg. Put another piece of bread on the top.

Serve.

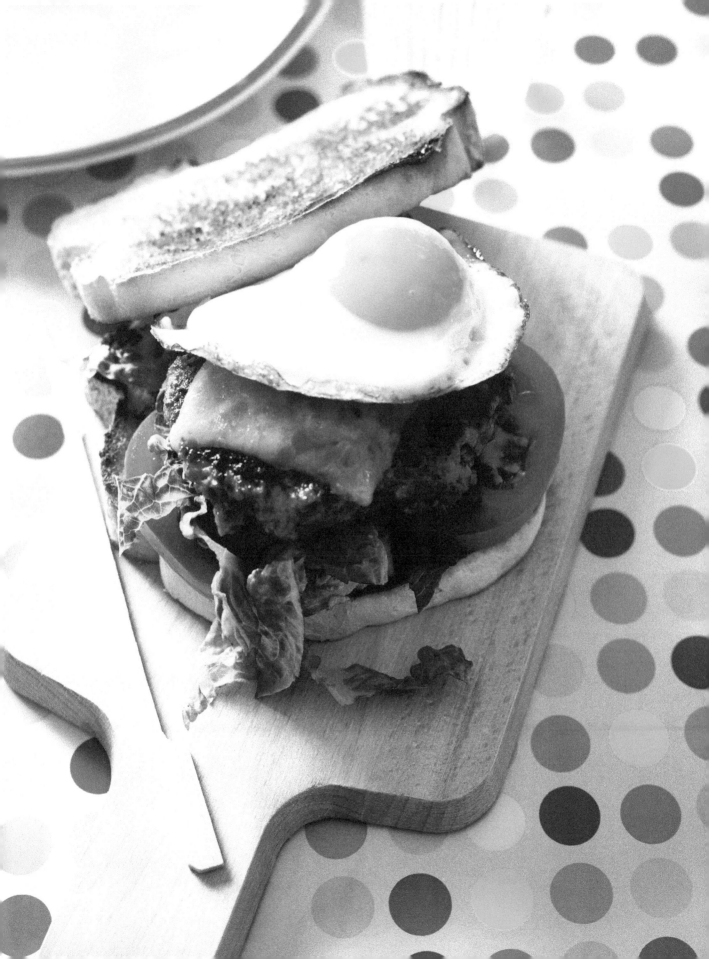

Lamb stew

Serves 6

1 tbsp olive oil

1kg lamb, diced

2 carrots, peeled, chopped

3 medium-sized potatoes, peeled, chopped into large cubes

¼ celery stick, diced

¼ cup parsley, finely chopped

½ cup chives, finely chopped

1 parsnip, diced

1 tsp rosemary, fresh

Salt

Black pepper

1 litre of chicken stock *(see recipe on page 20)*

2 tbsp butter

4 tbsp gluten-free cornflour

Place oil and lamb in a large saucepan over a medium heat and fry until lamb is browned.

Add carrot, potatoes, celery, parsley, chives, parsnip and rosemary as well as a seasoning of salt and pepper.

Pour in beef stock and bring to a boil, then simmer for 1 hour and 30 minutes.

Into a separate small saucepan, place the butter and cornflour and cook for about 1 minute. Add 1 cup of the liquid from the stew and whisk until it begins to thicken. Incorporate into the stew and simmer for a further 5 minutes, then season to taste.

Serve.

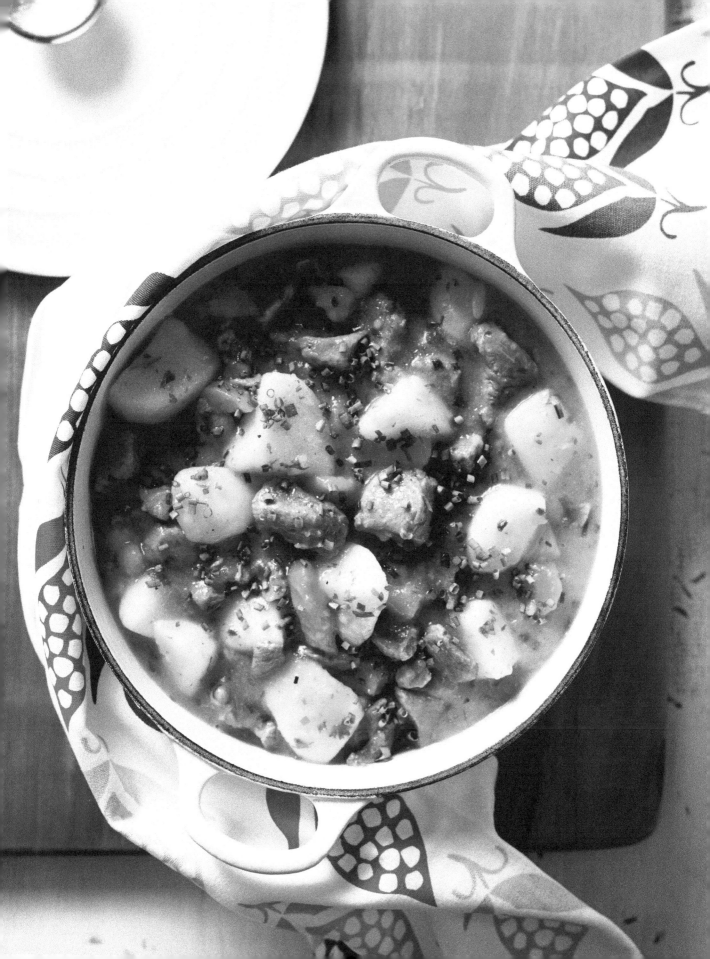

Lasagne

Serves 8

2 tbsp butter

4 tbsp gluten-free plain flour

½ tsp salt

¼ tsp black pepper

2 cups lactose-free milk

1 quantity spaghetti Bolognese sauce
(see recipe on page 62)

500g lactose-free cheese, grated

1 packet gluten-free lasagne sheets

Preheat oven to 180°C.

Melt the butter in a medium saucepan. Add flour, salt and pepper, and stir continuously over a medium heat for approx. 1 minute.

Next, pour in the milk and continue to stir constantly with a whisk until the sauce begins to thicken. When it thickens add 100g of the cheese and stir through. Season to taste and set aside.

Now assemble lasagne. In a 3 litre ovenproof dish, start with a layer of Bolognese sauce. Next, add a layer of white sauce. Now, a layer of lasagne sheets. Repeat this process until all ingredients have been used, ending with a layer of white sauce.

Cover with aluminium foil and place in the oven for 45 minutes. Take out and discard foil.

Cover with remaining grated cheese and return to the oven for a further 15 minutes until golden brown.

Serve.

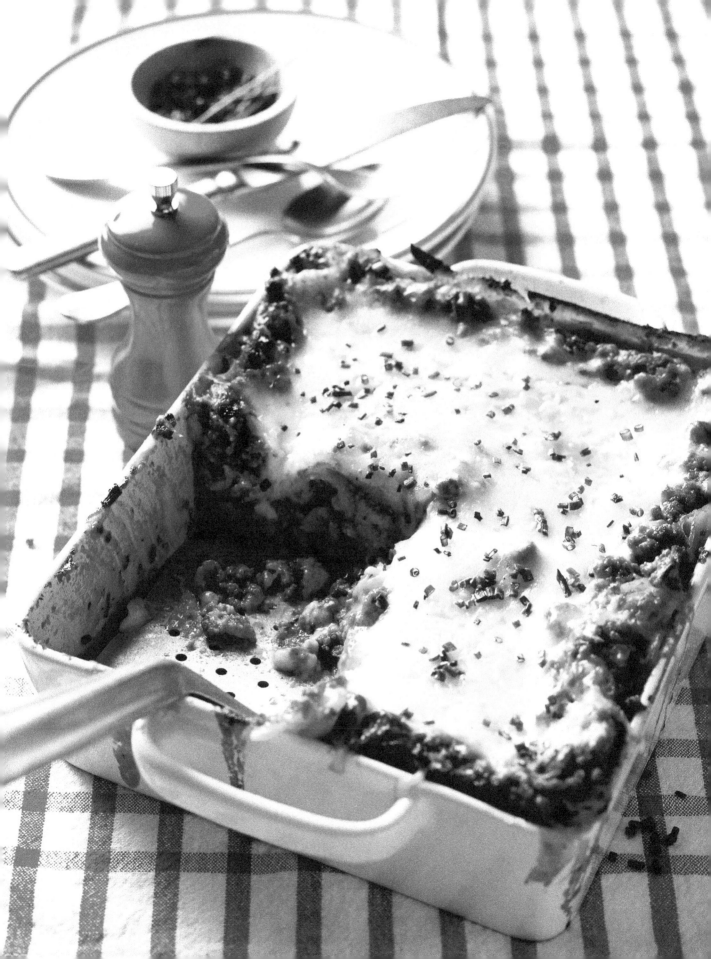

Mini pizzas

Makes 10

½ tbsp dried gluten-free yeast

¾ cup warm water

1 tsp dextrose powder

2½ cups gluten-free plain flour

¾ tsp salt

2 tbsp olive oil

¾ cup tomato paste

2 chicken thigh fillets, cooked and shredded

1 capsicum, diced

½ pineapple, diced

1 punnet cherry tomatoes, halved

400g lactose-free cheese, grated

Place dried yeast, warm water and dextrose powder in a small mixing bowl and stir well. Set aside until it becomes frothy.

In a separate large mixing bowl combine the flour and salt.

Make a hole in the middle of the flour and pour in the oil and yeast mixture. Using a fork, ensure mixture is well combined.

Next, lightly flour a bench and turn out the mixture. Knead well for 5 minutes.

Place back into the bowl and keep covered in a warm place to rise for approx. 25 minutes.

Preheat oven to 180°C.

Turn the dough back out onto the bench and separate into 10 pieces. Roll into pizza shapes 1 cm thick and place on a well-oiled baking tray.

Spread tomato paste on the base of the pizzas.

Next, cover with chicken, capsicum, pineapple, cherry tomatoes and finally the cheese.

Place in oven to cook until the pizza bases are golden brown approx. 20–25 minutes.

Serve.

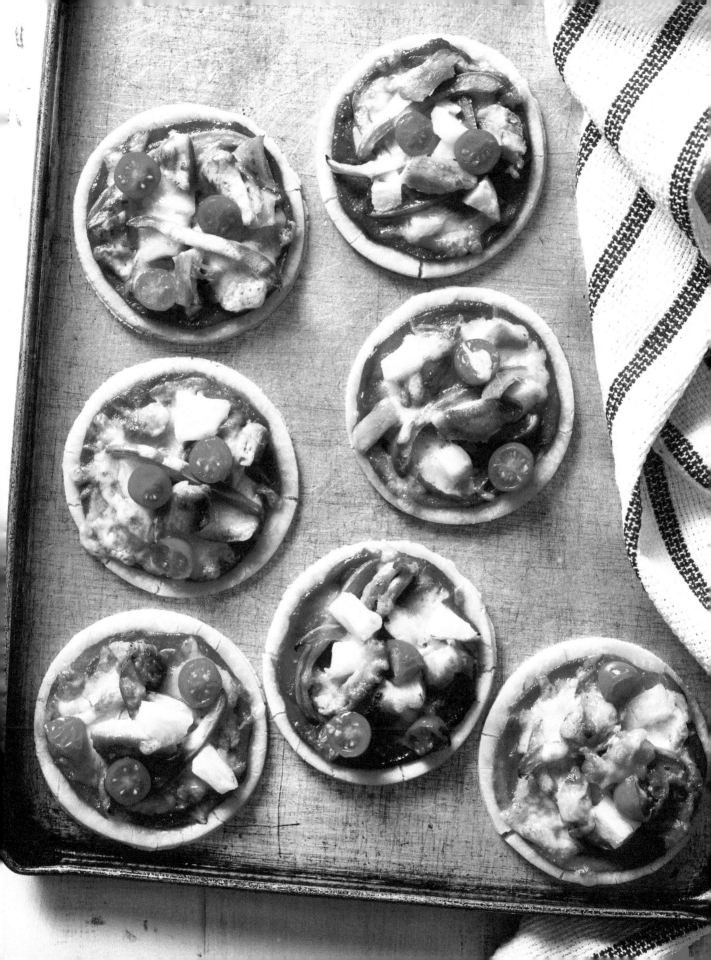

Moussaka

Serves 8

Olive oil

2 large eggplants, sliced thinly

1 cup chives, finely chopped

750g lamb mince

250g beef mince

2 tsp salt

1½ tbsp basil, fresh

½ tsp oregano, dried

¼ tsp allspice

¼ tsp ground cinnamon

2½ tbsp dextrose powder

350ml tomato puree

¼ cup tomato paste

2 tbsp butter

4 tbsp gluten-free plain flour

2 cups lactose-free milk

450g lactose-free cheese, grated

Salt

Ground black pepper

Preheat oven to 180°C.

Pour a liberal amount of oil into a large frying pan and fry the eggplant for 2–3 minutes on each side. Place the eggplant onto absorbent paper and set aside.

Next, pour a small amount of oil into a large saucepan and add the chives and minces. Cook until well browned.

Add salt, basil, oregano, allspice, cinnamon, dextrose, tomato puree and tomato paste. Incorporate well and allow to come to boil and then season to taste and set aside.

Melt the butter in a medium saucepan. Add, flour and stir continuously over medium heat for approx. 1 minute. Pour in the milk and continue to stir constantly with a whisk until the sauce begins to thicken. When it begins to thicken add 100g of the cheese and stir through. Season to taste. Set aside.

Now, in a 3 litre ovenproof dish, place a layer of eggplant followed by a layer of the meat sauce, then a layer of white sauce. Repeat this process finishing with a layer of white sauce. Sprinkle with remaining cheese.

Place in the oven and cook for 40–45 minutes or until golden brown.

Serve.

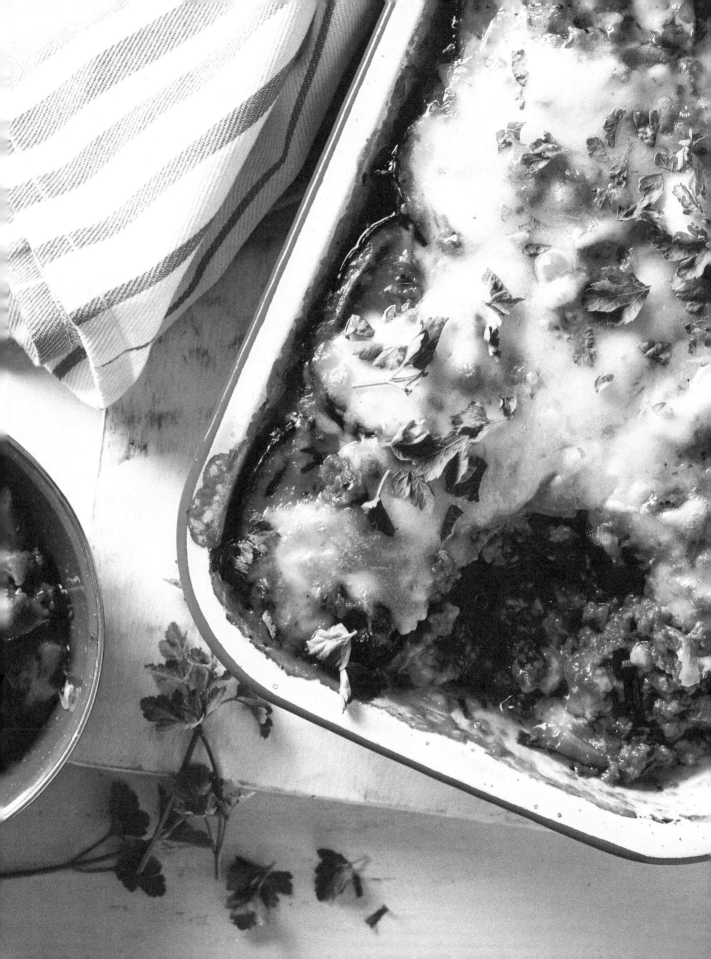

Oven spaghetti

Serves 6

1 tbsp olive oil

½ cup chives, chopped finely

1kg beef mince

1 cup beef stock
(see recipe on page 18)

1½ tsp salt

500g gluten-free spaghetti

½ cup gluten-free breadcrumbs

400g lactose-free cheese, grated

Preheat oven to 180°C.

Heat oil in a large saucepan and cook chives until wilted.

Add mince and salt and cook until browned. When meat is cooked add beef stock and season to taste.

Cook pasta according to packet instructions.

Into a 3 litre ovenproof dish, place a layer of the cooked pasta. Next, add a layer of the mince mixture. Sprinkle with bread crumbs and then a thin layer of cheese. Continue this way until all ingredients have been used, finishing with a spaghetti layer.

Sprinkle with the remaining cheese.

Place into the oven for 10–15 minutes or until it's golden brown on top.

Serve.

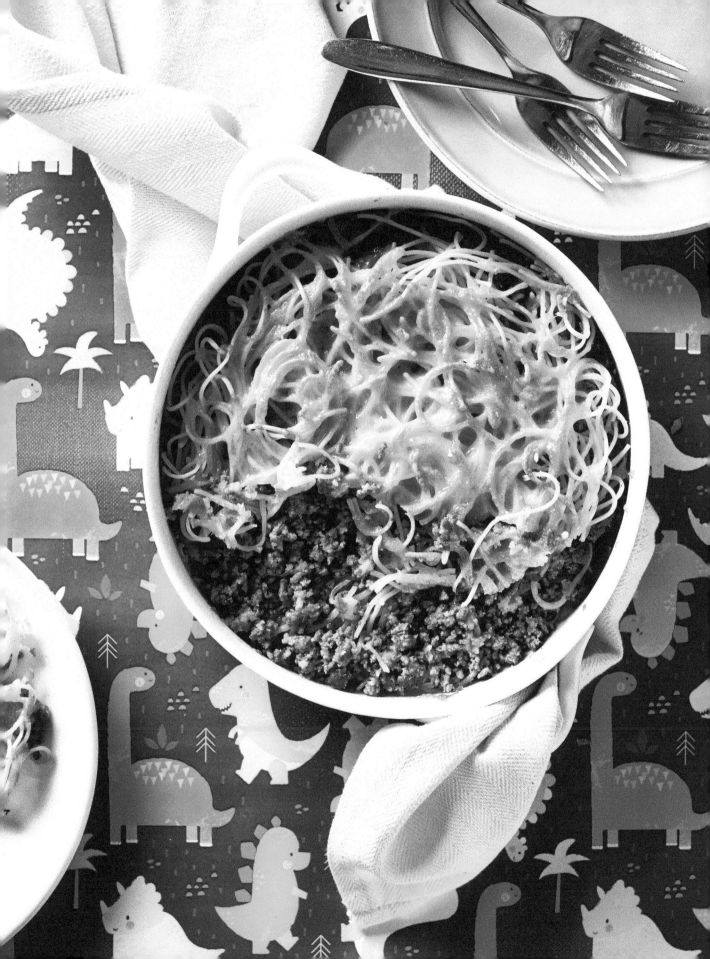

Peri peri chicken

Serves 4

½ cup parsley, chopped

¾ cup chives, chopped

1 small knob ginger, peeled

⅓ cup lemon juice

1 tsp dried chilli flakes

1½ tbsp canola oil

1½ tbsp rice wine vinegar

Pinch salt

Pinch black pepper

4 chicken marylands

Place parsley, chives, ginger, lemon juice, chili flakes, oil, vinegar, salt and pepper into a food processor. Process until ingredients are well combined.

Place chicken into a large mixing bowl and pour over the mixture. Be sure to coat the chicken well. Place in the fridge for at least 1¼ hours.

Preheat oven to 180°C.

Line a baking tray with baking paper.

Place chicken onto the tray, ensuring that any excess mixture is reapplied to the chicken.

Put chicken into the oven and cook for approx. 45–55 minutes, or until the chicken is golden brown and the juices run clear.

Serve.

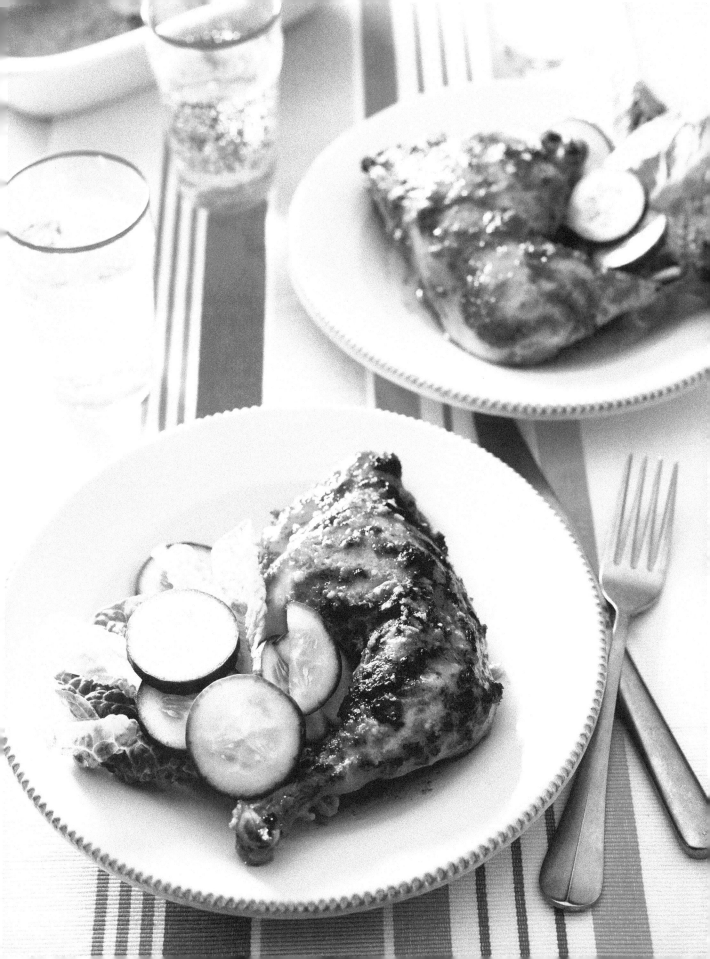

Pumpkin soup

Serves 6

2 tbsp olive oil

1.5 kg pumpkin, Jap, chopped

1 large potato, chopped

1 large carrot, chopped

½ tsp oregano, dried

½ cup chives, chopped

1¾ tsp salt

Ground black pepper

5 cups chicken stock
(see recipe on page 20)

1 cup of water

Heat oil in a large saucepan. Add the chopped vegetables, oregano, chives, salt and pepper and fry for 1 minute.

Pour in the stock and water and simmer for 1 hour, or until the vegetables are well cooked.

Using a stick blender, blend until smooth.

Simmer for a further 2 minutes, season to taste and serve.

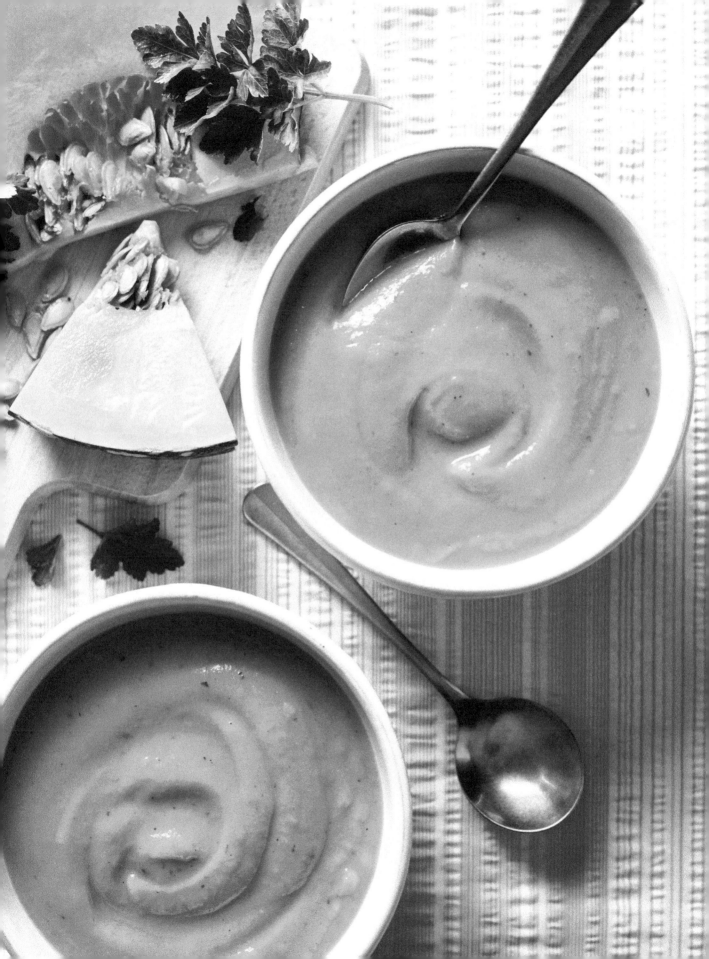

Red chicken

Serves 6

1kg chicken drumsticks

1 tbsp oregano, dried

⅓ cup chives, finely chopped

1 tsp salt

3 cups water

1 tsp butter

2 tbsp gluten-free cornflour

½ cup tomato paste

¼ cup dextrose powder

Place chicken, oregano, chives, salt and water into a large saucepan.

Bring chicken to boil, then simmer for approx. 30 minutes until chicken begins to fall off the bone.

In another small saucepan, melt the butter then add the corn flour and fry for approx. 30 seconds. Whisk in ½ cup of the chicken liquid until smooth. Take mixture off the stove and set aside.

When chicken is cooked, pour in the flour mixture and combine well. Return to a medium heat.

Add tomato paste and dextrose powder and stir through.

When tomato sauce begins to thicken, season to taste and take it off the heat.

Serve over pasta, rice and vegetables or mashed potato and vegetables.

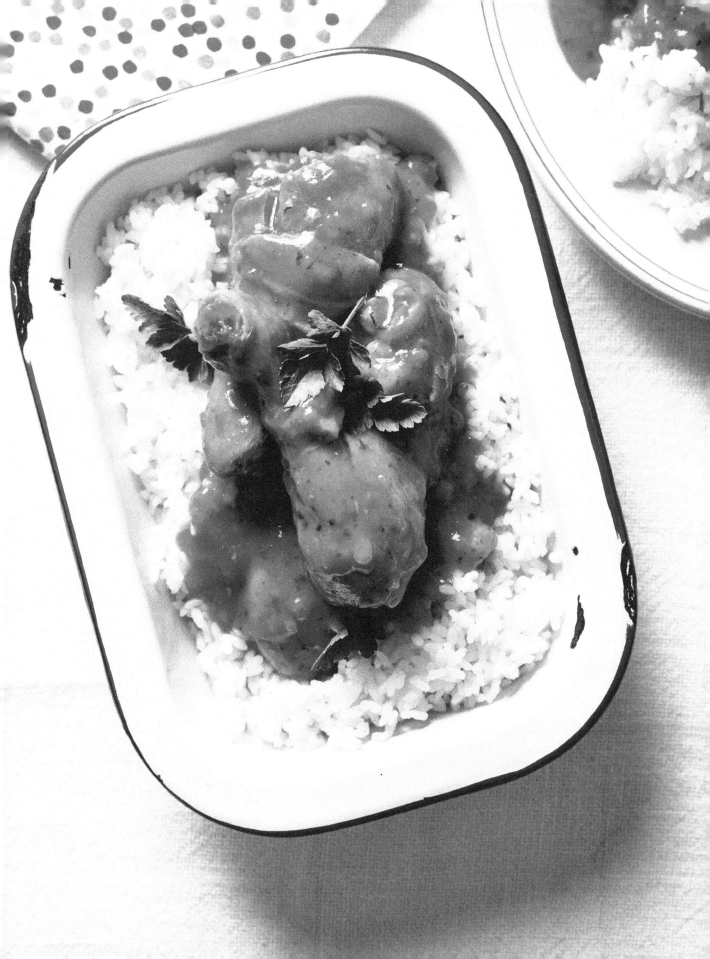

Red spaghetti and meatballs

Serves 6

1 quantity meatballs
(see recipe on page 66)

500g gluten-free pasta
(cooked as per packet instructions)

2 tbsp oil

1¼ cup chives, finely chopped

4 tbsp gluten-free plain flour

½ cup tomato paste

1½ cup water

1 tsp salt

2½ tbsp dextrose powder

Prepare meatballs and place in oven.

Cook pasta and set aside.

Place oil and chives into a large saucepan and fry over a medium heat for approx. 1 minute. Add the flour and continue cooking for a further 2 minutes.

Next, add the tomato paste and stir until well combined. Now add the water, salt and dextrose powder and continue cooking until the mixture begins to boil and thicken. The sauce should be thick enough to coat the pasta. Add extra seasoning to taste.

Pour in the cooked pasta and combine well.

Serve with meatballs.

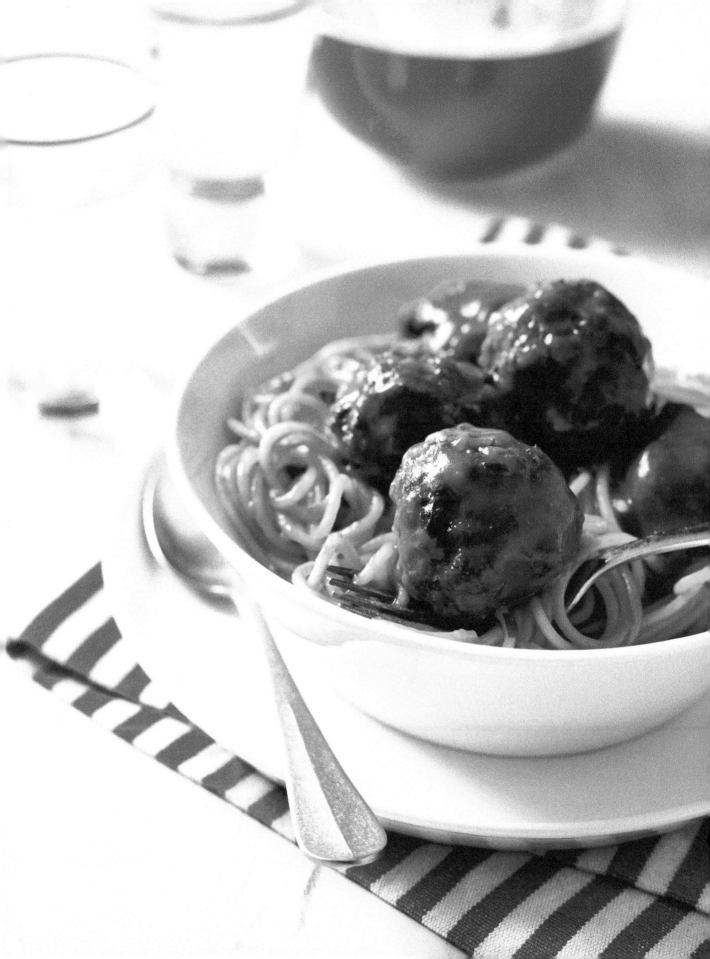

Rice paper rolls

Makes 12

1 quantity peri peri chicken *(see recipe on page 48)*

1 cucumber, common, thinly sliced

1 packet rice noodles (gluten free) *(prepare according to packet instructions)*

1 packet rice paper rolls (gluten free) *(prepare according to packet instructions)*

Pull the chicken off the bone and break into fine pieces in a large mixing bowl.

Into the same bowl, add the rice noodles and incorporate well.

Next, take a rice paper roll and place the chicken and noodle mix in the middle. Add desired amount of cucumber and roll up.

Set aside and repeat process.

Serve.

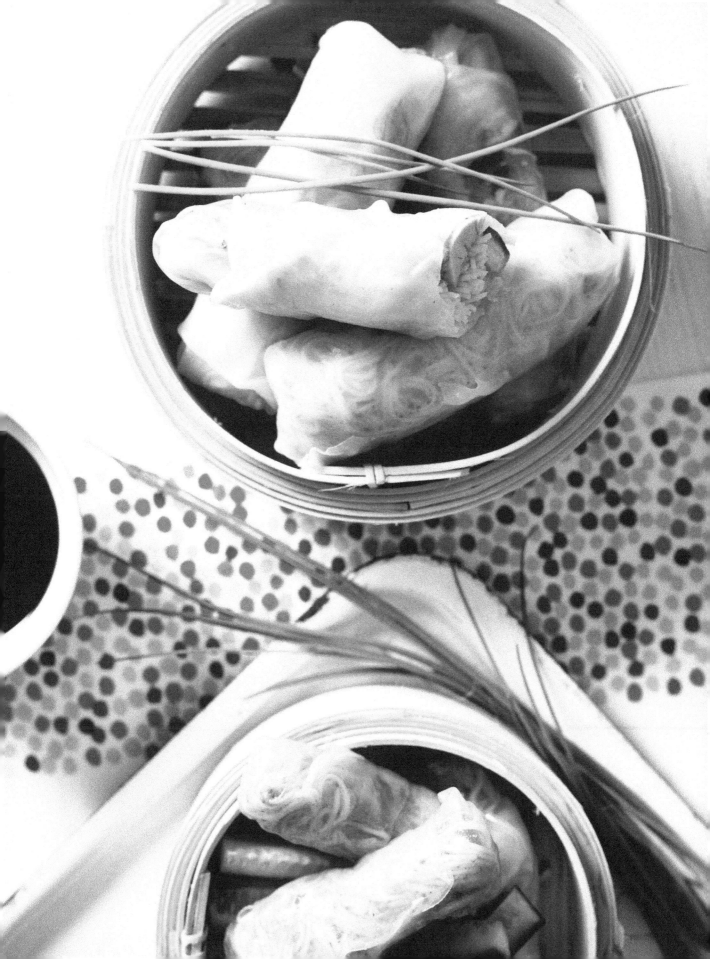

Roast lamb, veggies and gravy

Serves 6

1.5kg leg of lamb

3 sprigs rosemary

750g potatoes, chopped into medium pieces

250g carrots, chopped into large pieces

250g parsnips, chopped into large pieces

500g pumpkin, Jap, chopped into large pieces

Olive oil

1 tbsp salt

1 tsp butter

2 tbsp gluten-free plain flour

½ cup water

Preheat oven to 180°C.

Using a knife, make lots of little incisions in the leg of lamb. Into each incision stuff a leaf of rosemary.

Next, liberally coat the lamb with olive oil and salt. Place in a roasting dish and put in the oven. Cook for approx. 2 hours or until the meat is cooked through (check with a meat thermometer).

Place all of the chopped vegetables into a large mixing bowl and coat well with olive oil and salt. Place vegetables into a separate roasting dish and place in the oven for approx. 1 hour and 30 minutes or until well cooked.

To make the gravy, melt the butter in a small saucepan and then add the flour. Cook for approx. 1 minute, then, using a whisk, stir continuously as you incorporate the meat pan juices and water. Bring to the boil and set aside.

Serve.

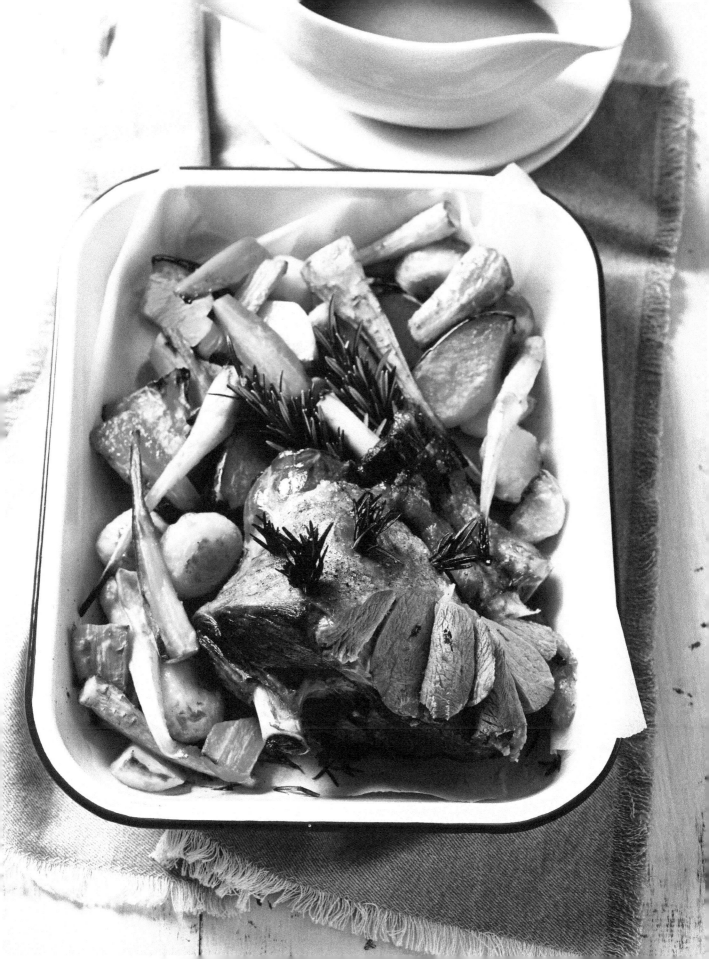

Savoury rice

Serves 6

1 tbsp olive oil

1 large carrot, chopped

¼ cup peas, thawed

½ cob of corn, de-hulled

¼ cup parsley, chopped finely

1 bunch spring onions (green tops only)

1kg beef mince

1½ cups white rice

3½ cups water

1½ tsp salt

½ tsp allspice

¼ tsp dried chili flakes

Place oil, carrot, peas, corn kernels, parsley and spring onions into a large saucepan over medium heat and sauté.

Add mince to the saucepan and brown well.

Pour in rice, water, salt, allspice and chilli flakes.

Bring to the boil then simmer for approx. 25 minutes or until rice is cooked. Stir occasionally and add seasoning to taste.

Serve.

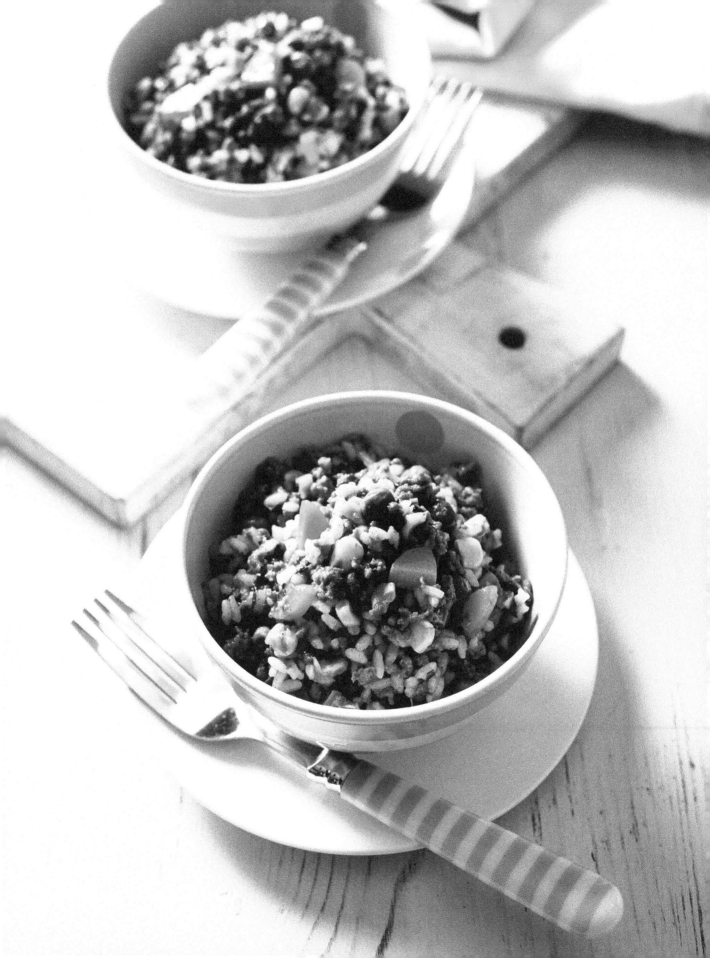

Spaghetti Bolognese

Serves 6

600g gluten-free pasta

750g beef mince

1½ tsp salt

1 tbsp parsley, chopped finely

1 tbsp oregano, dried

½ cup chives, chopped finely

1 tin whole peeled tomatoes

¼ cup water

½ small carrot, chopped

3½ tbsp dextrose powder

½ cup tomato paste

Bring a large saucepan of water to the boil and season with salt. Cook pasta according to packet instructions.

Place mince, salt, parsley, oregano and chives into a large saucepan, and cook until browned.

Next, place tinned tomatoes, water and carrot in a blender and puree.

Pour tomato mixture into the mince and simmer for approx. 10 minutes.

Finally, incorporate the dextrose powder and tomato paste. Bring to the boil and simmer for a further 15 minutes. Add extra water if required. Season to taste.

Spoon the meat sauce over the pasta and sprinkle with lactose-free cheese (optional).

Serve.

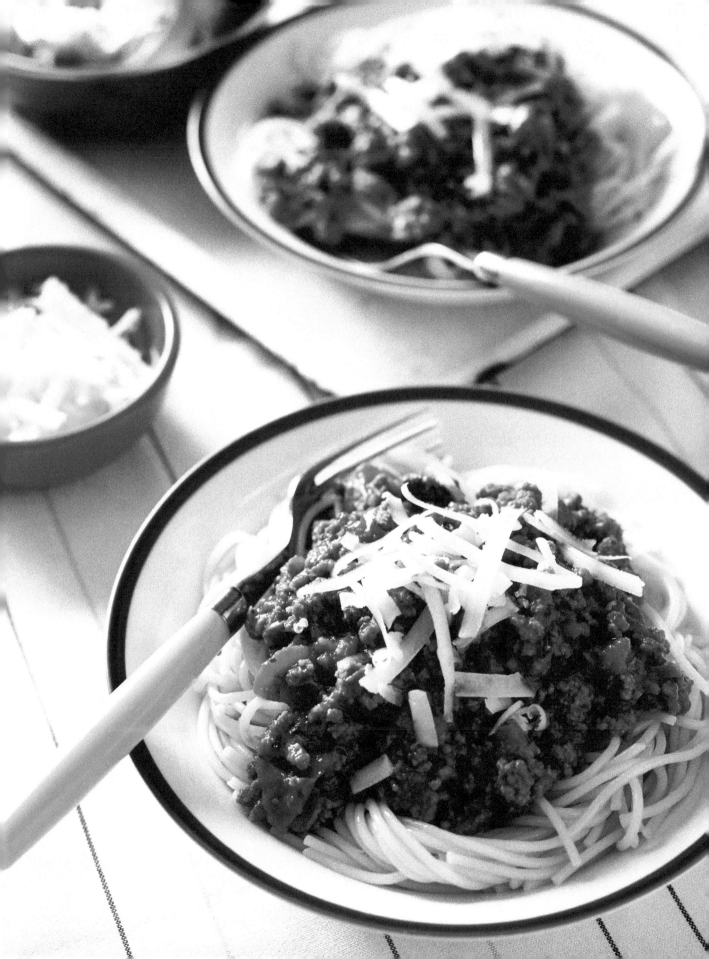

Stuffed capsicums

Serves 6

500g beef mince

1¼ cup ham hock salt brined; discard rind and finely dice

1¼ cup chives, finely chopped

¼ cup parsley, finely chopped

1 cup white rice, partly cooked

2 tsp salt

¼ tsp pepper

1 egg

6 capsicums, red or green

4 cups water

2 tbsp butter

4 tbsp gluten-free cornflour

½ tsp paprika

¾ cup tomato paste

1½ tbsp dextrose powder

Place mince, ham hock, chives, parsley, rice, salt, pepper and egg into a large mixing bowl. Combine well with your hands.

Cut the stem end off of each capsicum and pull out all of the seeds.

Next, stuff the mince mixture inside the capsicums, being careful to only fill them ¾ of the way to the top.

Place the capsicums in a large saucepan and add 3 cups water. The water should not completely cover the capsicums.

Place a lid on the saucepan and simmer for approx. 45 minutes.

Next, into a small saucepan place butter, paprika and cornflour and cook for 1 minute. Add tomato paste, dextrose and 1 cup of water, cook until begins to thicken. Pour tomato mixture into capsicums and combine well. This is to give the capsicums a lovely sweet sauce.

Cook for a further 5 minutes, season to taste, then allow to sit for another 5 minutes with the heat off.

Serve.

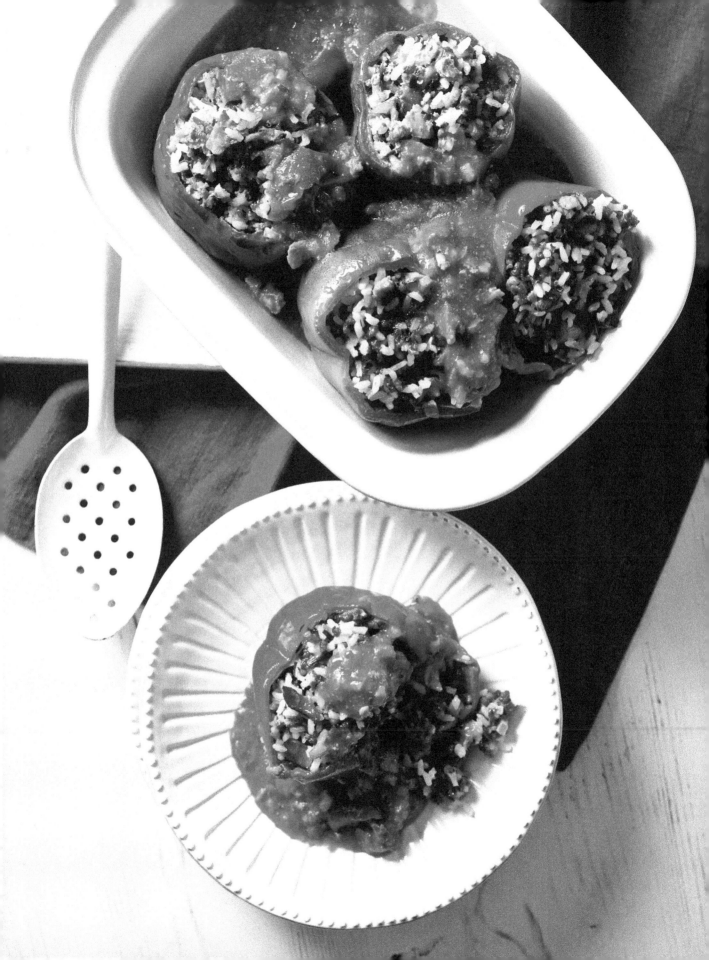

Meatballs and salsa dip

Makes 18

500g beef mince

¼ cup chives, chopped finely

1 tbsp parsley, chopped finely

½ tbsp mint, chopped finely

2 tbsp gluten-free plain flour

1 egg, beaten

1/3 cup parmesan cheese or lactose-free tasty cheese, grated

½ tsp salt

Pepper, pinch

1 quantity salsa
(see recipe on page 67)

Preheat oven to 180°C.

Place mince, chives, parsley, mint, flour, egg, cheese, salt and pepper into a large mixing bowl and combine well.

Take small handfuls of the mixture and roll into balls, then place on a lined baking tray.

Cook for approx. 25–30 minutes, ensuring that you turn the meatballs to get an even, golden brown.

Serve with salsa.

Tomato salsa

1 punnet cherry tomatoes

½ cup chives, roughly chopped

½ tsp salt

½ tsp dried chilli flakes

1 tbsp lemon juice

2 tsp dextrose powder

Place all ingredients in a food processor and blend well.

Pour into a small saucepan and bring to a boil. Simmer for 8–10 minutes or until reduced to desired consistency. Season to taste.

Serve.

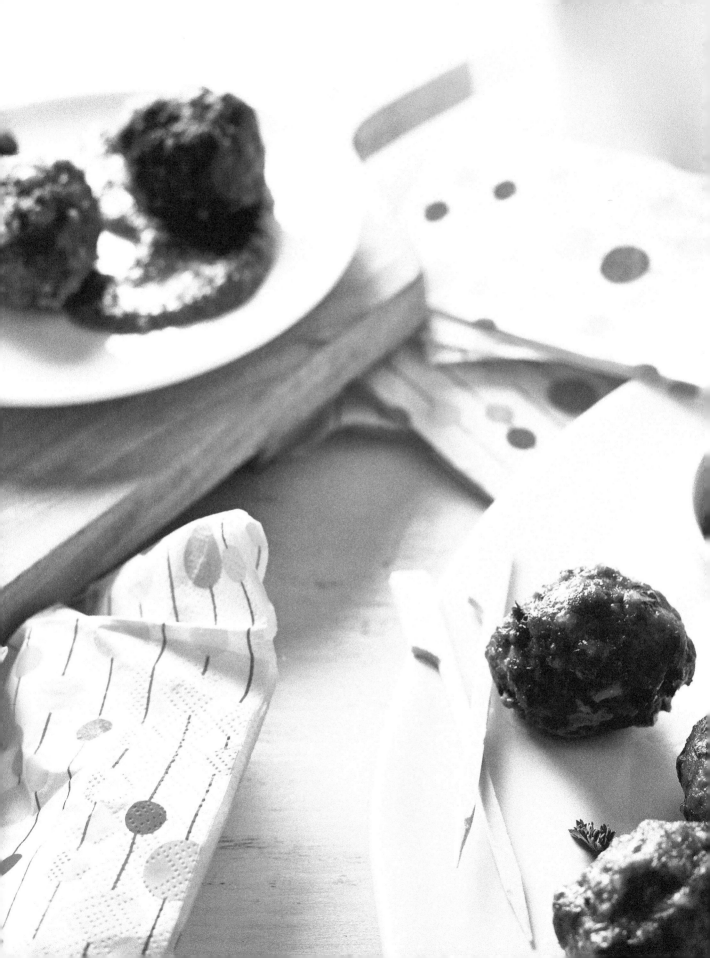

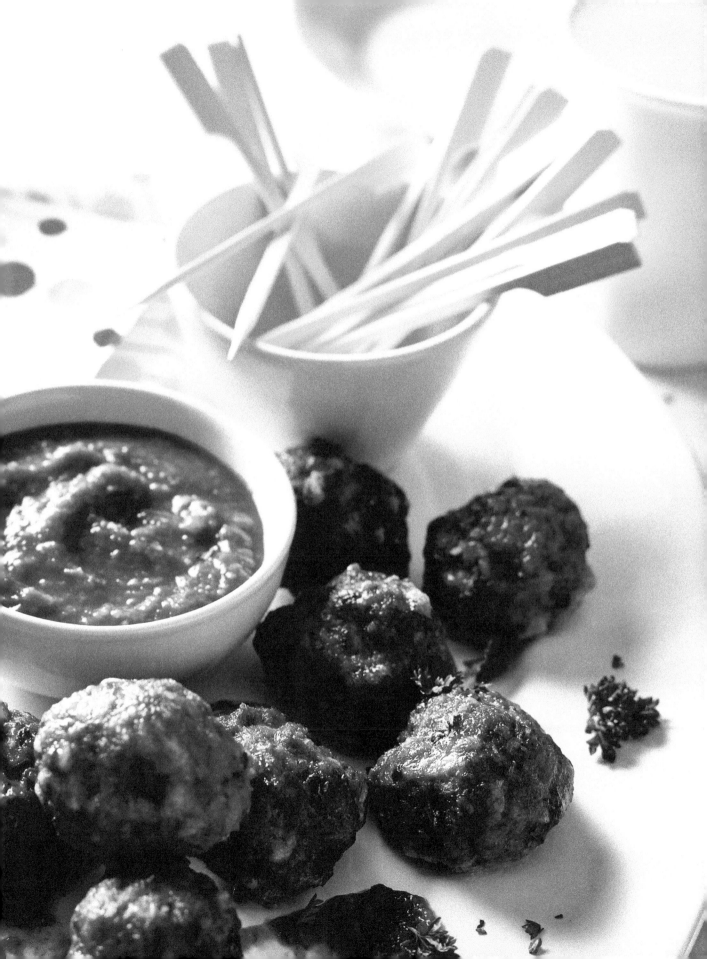

Meat sauce and rice

Serves 4

1 tbsp olive oil

1 cup chives, finely chopped

500g beef mince

½ tsp salt

1 tsp paprika

2 tbsp gluten-free plain flour

1½ cups beef stock
(see recipe on page 18)

1½ cups rice
(cook according to packet instructions)

Heat oil in a large saucepan and cook chives until wilted.

Add mince and cook until brown. When meat is browned add salt, paprika and flour and cook for a further 1 minute. Next, pour in beef stock and allow to boil and thicken. Serve over cooked rice.

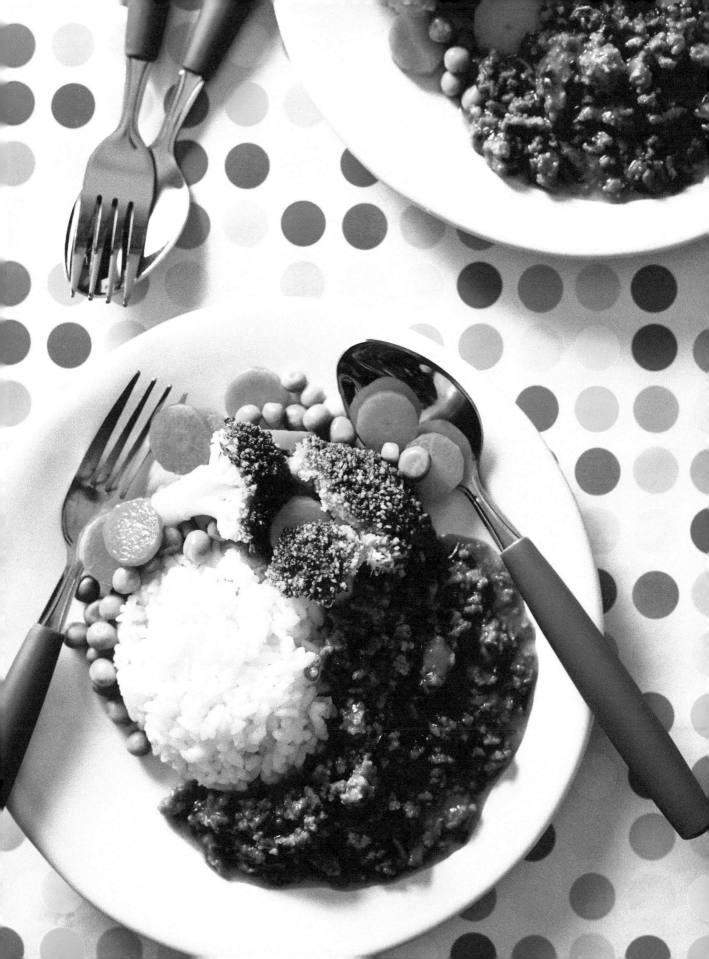

Tomato, cheese and chive muffins

Makes 8

1⅓ cups lactose-free cheese, grated

16 cherry tomatoes, halved

½ cup chives, finely chopped

2½ tbsp parsley, finely chopped

⅔ cup lactose-free milk

2 eggs, beaten

¼ tsp salt

Pepper, pinch

1½ cups gluten-free self-raising flour

3 tbsp canola oil

Preheat oven to 180°C.

Combine cheese, cherry tomatoes, chives, parsley, milk, eggs, salt and pepper in a large mixing bowl.

Next, add the flour and incorporate well.

Using a pastry brush, coat the holes of a muffin tin with the oil.

Using a spoon, fill each hole about halfway.

Place in the oven and cook for approx. 18–20 minutes or until a skewer comes out clean when inserted in the middle.

Serve.

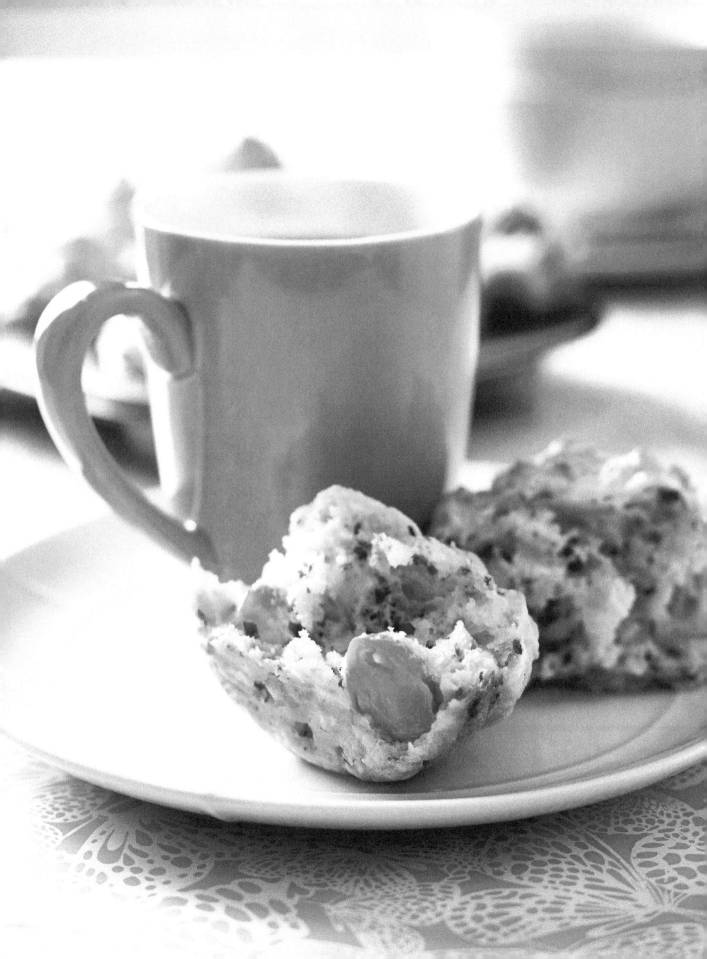

Tuna mornay

Serves 4

1 × 185g tin of tuna in oil

¼ cup chives, finely chopped

1 tbsp gluten-free plain flour

½ tsp salt

1 tsp paprika

1¼ cups lactose-free milk

1 packet gluten-free pasta *(cook according to packet instructions)*

Add tuna and chopped chives to a medium saucepan.

Once the chives have wilted, add the flour, salt and paprika.

Continuously stirring, allow the mixture to fry off (we want the flour to cook).

When the mixture has cooked for about 30–45 seconds, pour in the milk.

Stir mixture constantly until it starts to thicken and simmer. Pour over pasta and combine well. Season to taste.

Take off heat and serve. For a variation, serve sauce with rice and vegetables.

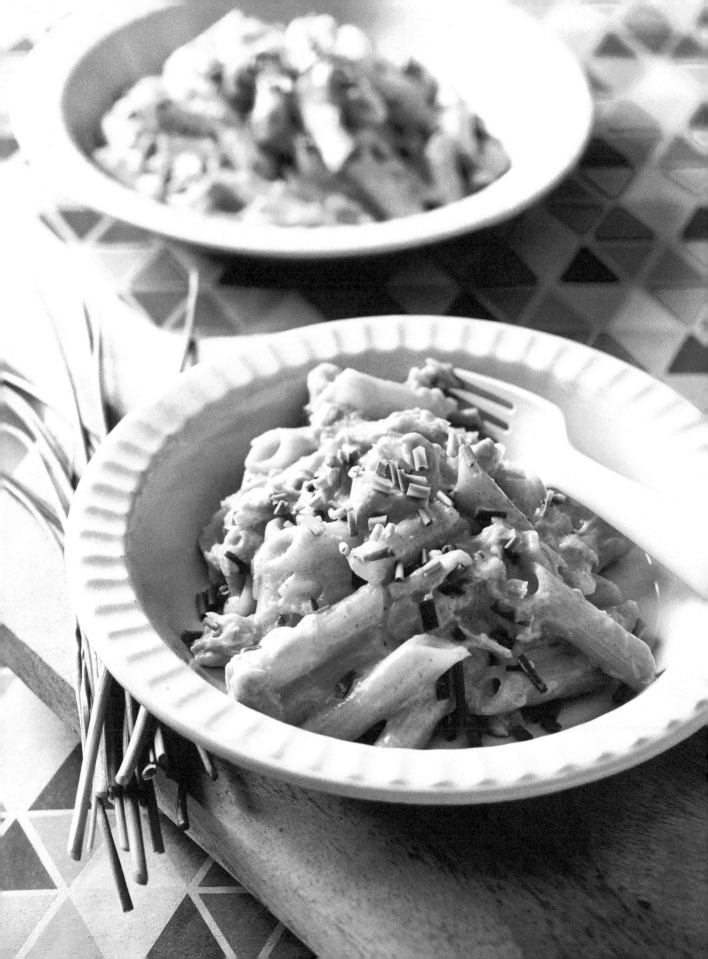

Tuna salad

Serves 2

95g tin tuna in oil

½ punnet cherry
tomatoes, halved

1 cucumber, common,
diced thickly

3 leaves, cos lettuce

¼ red capsicum, thinly
sliced

½ tbsp chives, finely
chopped

3 hard-boiled eggs, peeled
and diced thickly

Salt to taste

Into a salad bowl, place the tuna that has been half drained (ensure that you break the tuna up well, with a fork).

Next, add the cherry tomatoes, cucumber, lettuce, capsicum, chives, eggs and salt.

Combine well and serve.

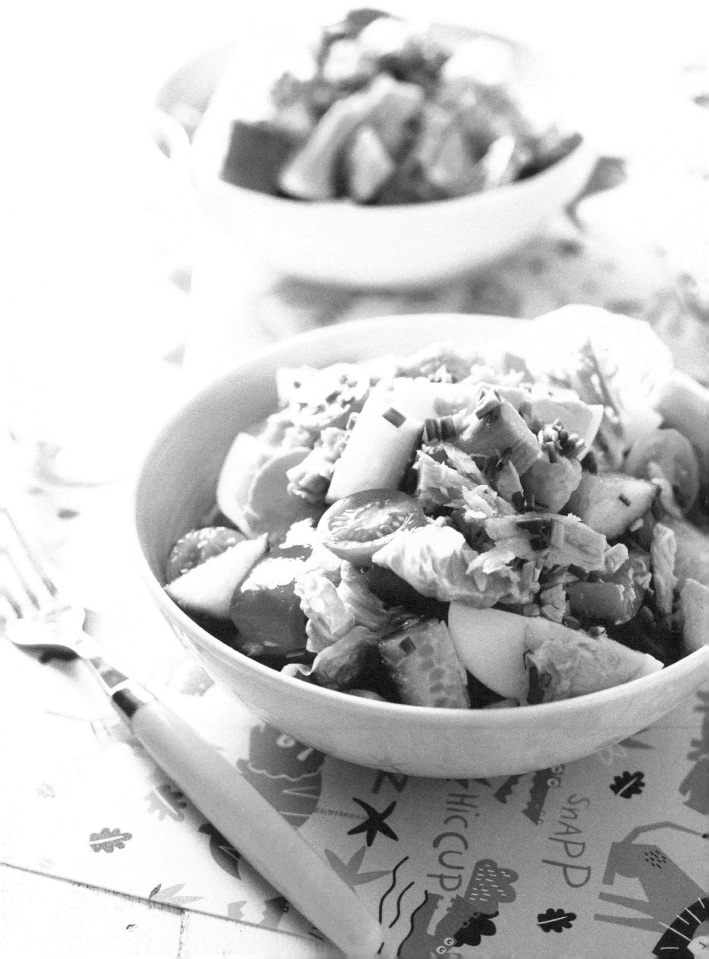

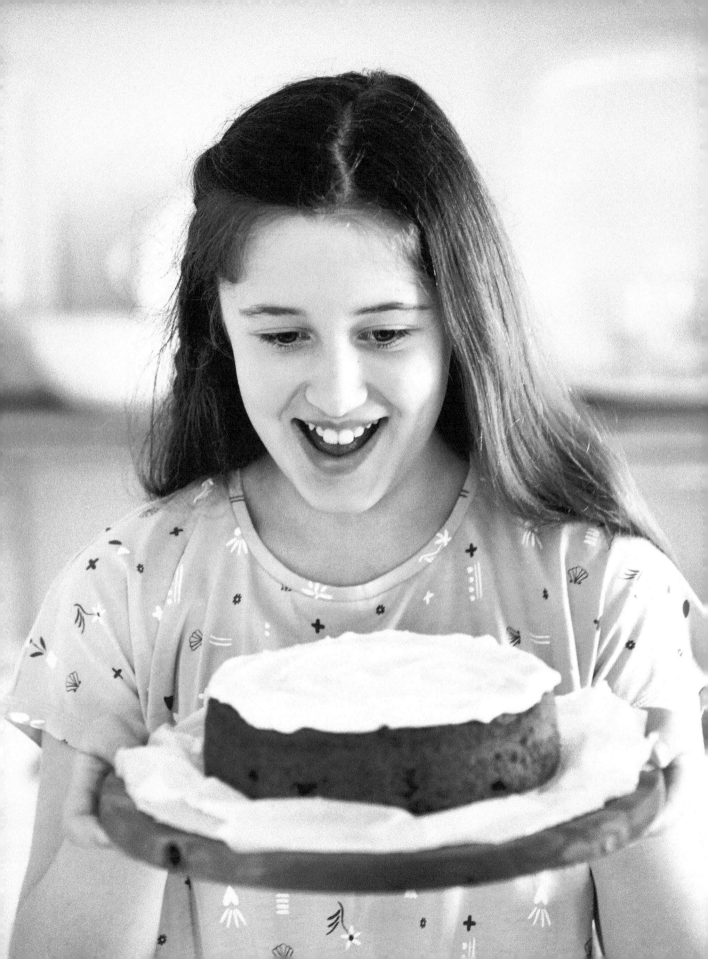

SWEET

Anzac biscuits

Makes 16

1¾ cups gluten-free plain flour

1 cup quinoa flakes

¼ cup coconut, shredded, dried

½ tsp ground cinnamon

½ tsp sugar-free pure vanilla extract

1 tbsp dextrose powder

125g butter

¾ cup rice malt syrup

1½ tbsp boiling hot water

½ tsp gluten-free bicarb soda

Preheat oven to 180°C.

Place flour, quinoa flakes, coconut, cinnamon, vanilla and dextrose powders into a large mixing bowl. Combine ingredients well and set aside.

Place the butter and rice malt syrup into a small saucepan on a low heat until butter has melted.

In a separate small mixing bowl, place boiling water and bicarb soda, and mix until dissolved. Once dissolved, put bicarb mixture in the saucepan with the rice malt syrup.

When rice malt mixture begins to bubble, add to flour mixture and combine well.

Place tablespoon-sized scoops on a tray lined with baking paper.

Cook for approx. 15–20 minutes until golden brown.

Cool and serve.

Chocolate biscuits

Makes 16

125g butter

½ cup rice malt syrup

2 cups gluten-free plain flour

½ cup dextrose powder

¼ cup pure cocoa powder

1½ tbsp boiling water

½ tsp gluten-free bicarb soda

Preheat oven to 170°C.

Place butter and rice malt syrup into a small saucepan over a low heat.

Combine flour, dextrose and cocoa powder in a large mixing bowl.

In a separate small mixing bowl, combine the boiling water and bicarb soda.

When butter has melted, pour bicarb mixture into saucepan.

When mixture begins to bubble, pour into dry ingredients and stir well.

Place tablespoon-sized scoops of the mixture onto a baking paper-lined baking tray.

Place in oven and cook for approx. 18–20 minutes.

Serve.

Gingernut biscuits

Makes 16

125g butter

½ cup rice malt syrup

1¾ cups gluten-free plain flour

1 tsp gluten-free bicarb soda

1 tbsp ground ginger

1 tsp ground cinnamon

½ cup dextrose powder

Preheat oven to 170°C.

Melt butter and rice malt syrup in a small saucepan and stir until combined.

In a large mixing bowl, combine the flour, bicarb soda, ginger, cinnamon and dextrose powder.

Next, pour butter mixture into the dry ingredients and incorporate well.

Place tablespoon-sized scoops of the mixture onto a baking paper-lined baking tray.

Place in oven for approx. 18–20 minutes or until golden brown.

Serve.

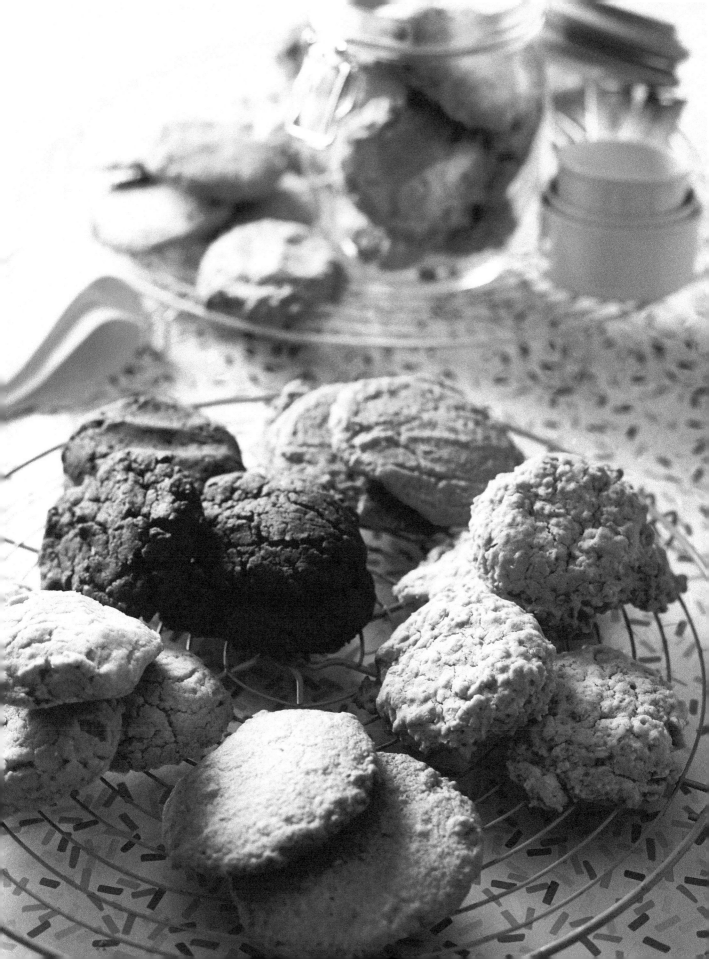

Shortbread biscuits

Makes 16

200g butter, chilled and diced

¾ cup dextrose powder

2 cups gluten-free plain flour

½ tsp xanthan gum

½ tsp gluten-free bicarb soda

Preheat oven to 170°C.

Place butter and dextrose powder into a food processor and mix until well combined.

Add flour, xanthan gum and bicarb soda on a medium speed and process until mixture resembles wet breadcrumbs.

Turn out onto a lightly floured surface and knead until the mixture comes together like a dough.

Roll dough out to about 2cm thickness and cut with cookie cutters.

Place on a lined baking tray and cook in the oven for approx. 20–25 minutes, or until golden brown.

Serve.

Vanilla biscuits

Makes 16

125g butter

1 tsp sugar-free pure vanilla extract

½ cup rice malt syrup

2 cups gluten-free plain flour

½ cup dextrose powder

1½ tbsp boiling water

½ tsp gluten-free bicarb soda

Preheat oven to 170°C.

Place butter, vanilla and rice malt syrup into a small saucepan over a low heat.

Combine flour and dextrose powder in a large mixing bowl.

In a separate small mixing bowl, combine the boiling water and bicarb soda.

When the butter has melted, pour the bicarb mixture into the saucepan.

When mixture begins to bubble, pour into dry ingredients and stir well.

Place tablespoon-sized scoops of the mixture onto a baking paper-lined baking tray.

Place in oven and cook for approx. 18–20 minutes.

Serve.

Baked custard

Serves 6

3 eggs

1 cup dextrose powder

1 tsp sugar-free pure vanilla extract

1 cup lactose-free milk

300ml lactose-free thickened cream

Ground nutmeg (optional)

Preheat oven to 160°C.

Whisk eggs and dextrose powder in a large mixing bowl until well combined.

Add vanilla, milk and cream and continue to whisk until all ingredients are incorporated.

Pour into individual ramekins, only filling 2/3 full, then sprinkle with nutmeg (optional).

Put the ramekins in a 3 litre oven dish and pour boiling water halfway up the sides of the ramekins.

Place in oven and bake for approx. 45–50 minutes or until there is only a slight wobble to the custard.

Cool and serve.

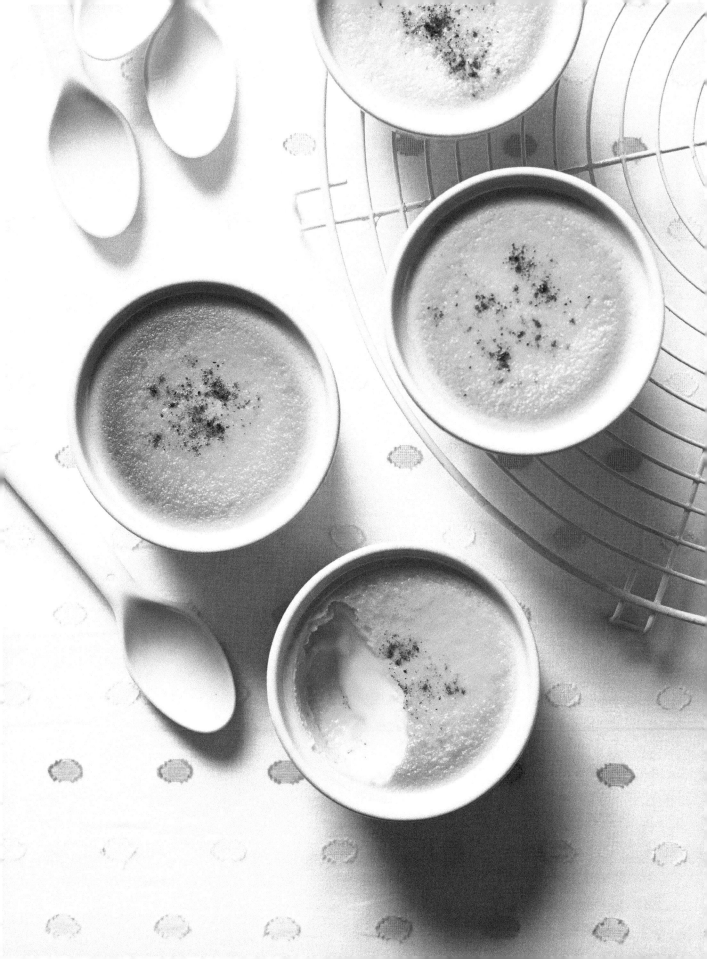

Banana and blueberry cake

Serves 10

1½ cups gluten-free self-raising flour, sifted

½ tsp gluten-free bicarb soda

1½ cups dextrose powder

1 egg, beaten

1 tsp sugar-free pure vanilla extract

¼ cup lactose-free milk

2 bananas, medium, mashed (just ripened)

50g butter, melted

1 punnet blueberries

Icing

250g lactose-free cream cheese

¼ cup lactose-free milk

⅓ cup dextrose powder

1 orange, rind only

Preheat oven to 170°C.

Into a medium mixing bowl place flour, bicarb soda and dextrose powder and set aside.

In a separate large mixing bowl combine egg, vanilla, milk and mashed bananas.

Next, fold the flour mixture into the banana mixture and add the butter.

Finally, add the blueberries.

When well incorporated, place in a lined 19cm springform tin.

Cook for approx. 55–60 minutes, or until a skewer inserted in the middle comes out clean.

Set aside to cool.

Into a mixer place cream cheese, milk, dextrose powder and orange rind. Incorporate well until smooth consistency.

Finally, ice top of cake with icing mixture.

Serve.

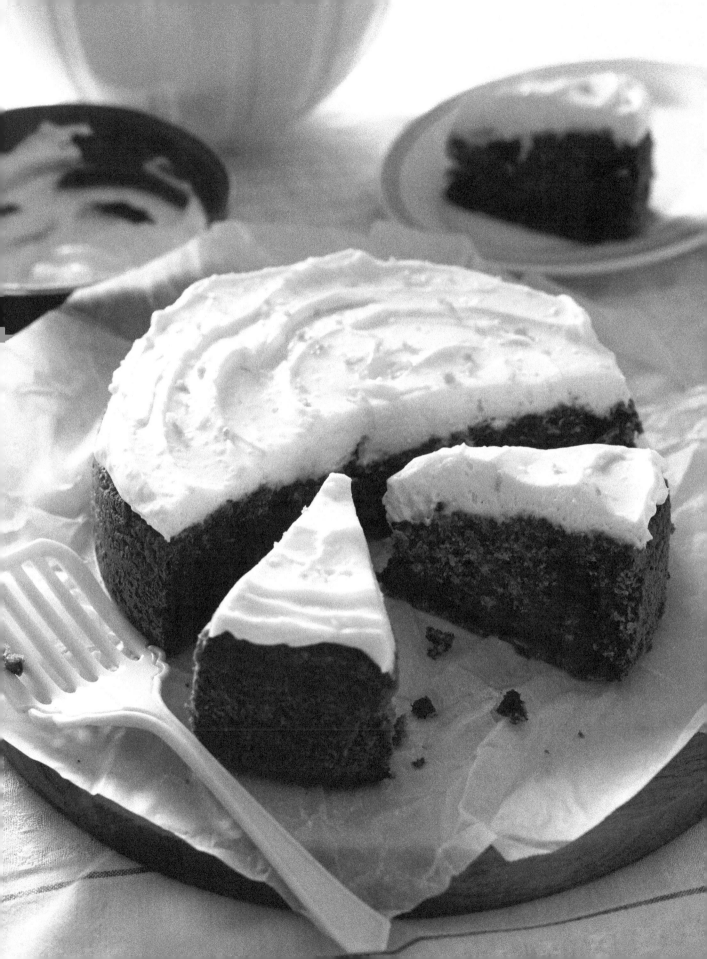

Banana milkshake

Serves 2

2 cups lactose-free milk

1 banana, peeled (just ripened)

1 scoop vanilla ice-cream
(see recipe on page 120)

4 tbsp rice malt syrup

Place the milk, banana, ice-cream and rice malt syrup in a blender.

Blend until smooth and serve.

Caramel milkshake

Serves 2

1 scoop vanilla ice-cream
(see recipe on page 120)

1 cup lactose-free milk

3 tbsp caramel sauce
(see recipe on page 107)

Place the ice-cream, milk and caramel sauce into a blender.

Blend on low until ingredients are well combined, then serve.

Chocolate milkshake

Serves 2

1 scoop vanilla ice-cream
(see recipe on page 120)

1 cup lactose-free milk

3 tbsps chocolate sauce
(see recipe on page 108)

Place the ice-cream, milk and chocolate sauce in a blender.

Blend on low until ingredients are well combined.

Serve.

Strawberry milkshake

Serves 2

1 scoop vanilla ice-cream
(see recipe on page 120)

1 cup lactose-free milk

½ punnet strawberries,
hulled

3 tbsp dextrose powder

Place the ice-cream, milk, dextrose powder and strawberries into a blender.

Blend on low until ingredients are well combined, then serve.

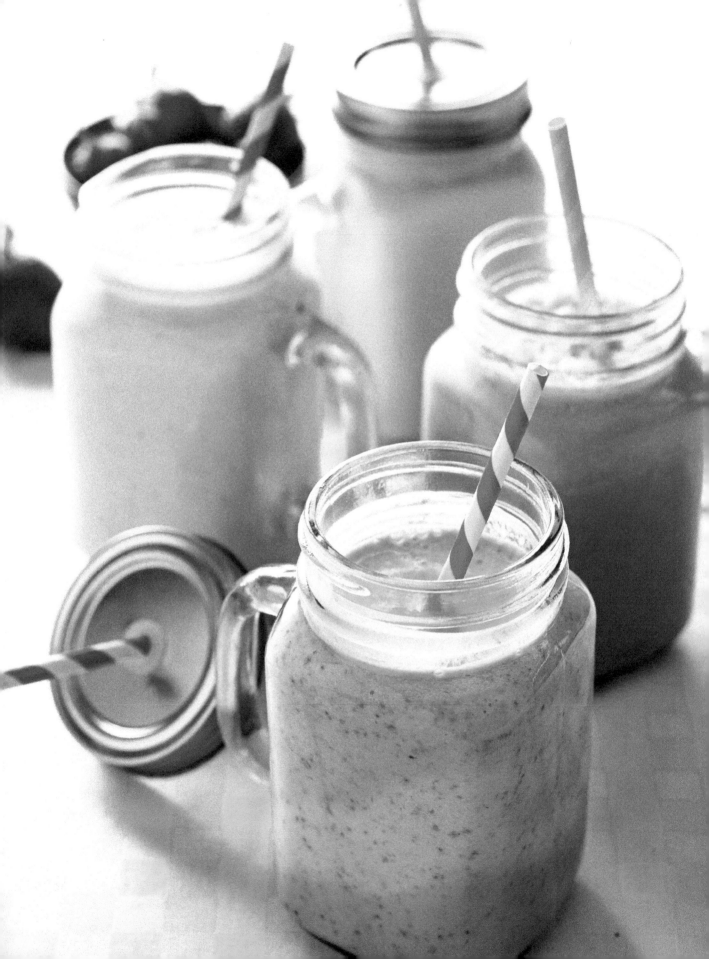

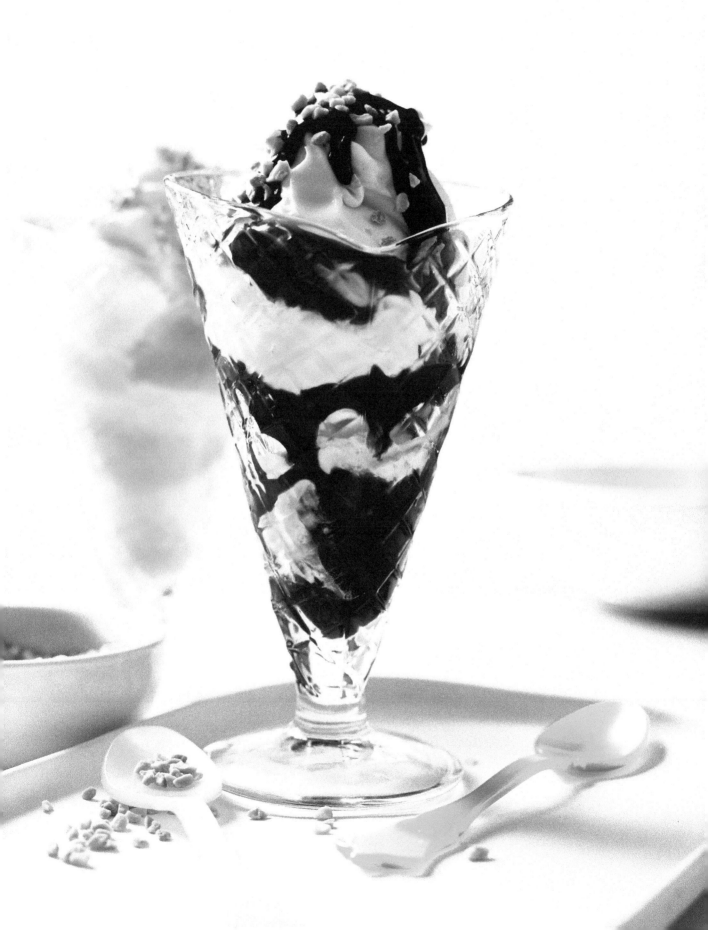

Caramel sundae

Serves 1

2 scoops vanilla ice-cream
(see recipe on page 120)

2 tbsps caramel sauce
(see recipe on page 107)

2 tbsp whipped cream
(see recipe on page 153)

1 tbsp peanuts, crushed

1 strawberry, halved

Place the ice-cream in a sundae glass.

Pour caramel sauce over the ice-cream.

Cover in whipped cream.

Sprinkle with peanuts and top with a strawberry.

Serve.

Chocolate sundae

Serves 1

2 scoops vanilla ice-cream
(see recipe on page 120)

2 tbsps chocolate sauce
(see recipe on page 108)

2 tbsp whipped cream
(see recipe on page 153)

1 tbsp peanuts, crushed

1 strawberry, halved

Place ice-cream in a sundae glass.

Pour chocolate sauce over the ice-cream.

Next, cover in whipped cream.

Sprinkle with peanuts and top with a strawberry.

Serve.

Banana split

Serves 1

1 banana, sliced in half lengthways (just ripened)

2 scoops vanilla ice-cream *(see recipe on page 120)*

2 tbsps chocolate sauce *(see recipe on page 108)*

1 tbsp crushed peanuts

Place banana halves in a dessert bowl.

Put 3 scoops of ice-cream on top of the banana.

Pour chocolate sauce over the ice-cream.

Finally, sprinkle with crushed peanuts.

Serve.

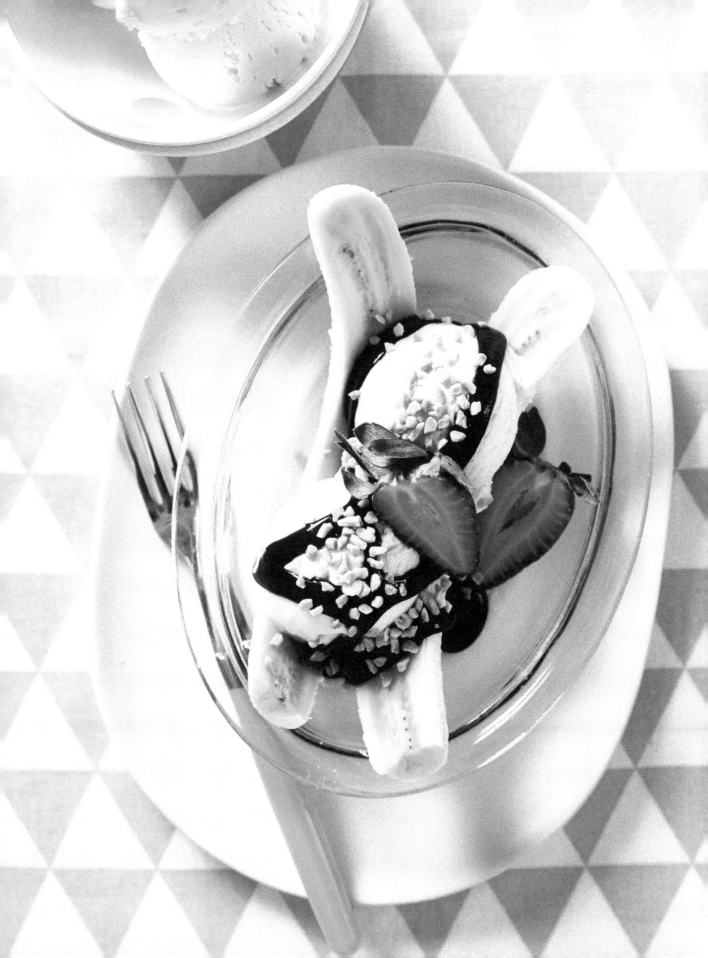

Blueberry crumble

Serves 8

2 punnets of blueberries

1¼ cups dextrose powder

½ cups gluten-free self-raising flour

½ cup quinoa flakes

70g butter, chilled

Preheat oven to 180°C

Place the blueberries and ¾ cup of dextrose powder into a medium saucepan.

Combine well and bring to the boil, and then simmer for approx. 5 minutes.

Pour blueberry mixture into a small baking dish and set aside.

Into a medium mixing bowl, place the flour, remaining dextrose powder, quinoa flakes and butter. Incorporate well with your hands until breadcrumb consistency. Sprinkle liberally over the blueberry mixture and place in the oven for 20–25 minutes or until golden brown on top.

Serve.

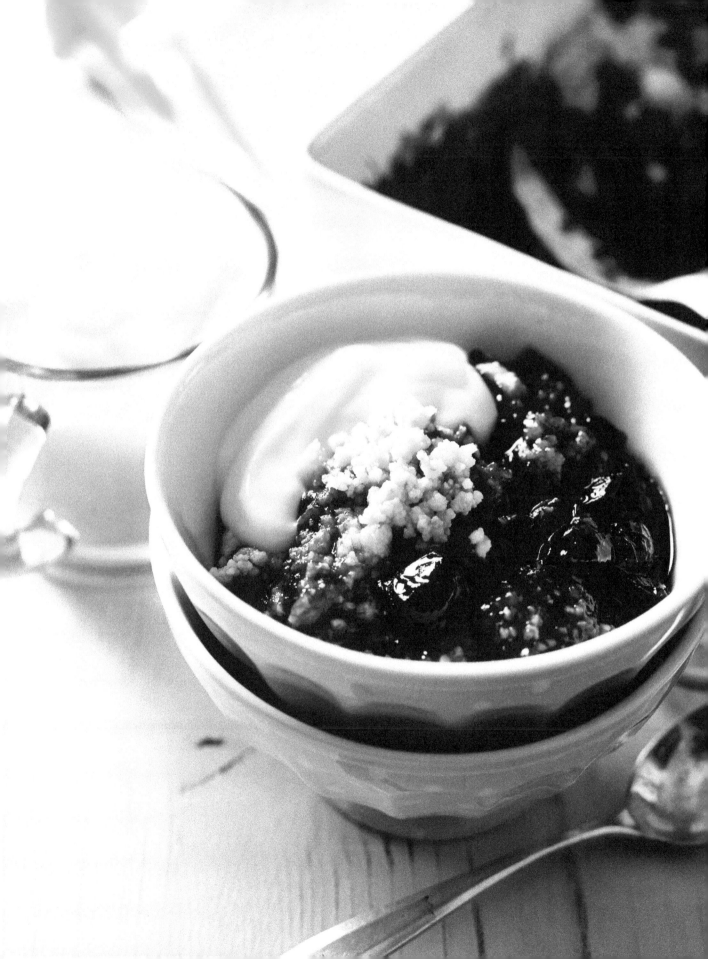

Custard

Serves 6

2 eggs

3 tbsp gluten-free cornflour

3 cups lactose-free milk

½ cup dextrose powder

1 tsp sugar-free pure vanilla extract

Whisk eggs, cornflour and milk together in a medium saucepan on a low to medium heat until smooth. Continue whisking until mixture begins to thicken.

When thickened, remove from heat and whisk in vanilla.

Serve.

Blueberry jam

Makes 1 jar

2 punnets of blueberries

2 tbsp lemon juice

1¼ cups dextrose powder

Place the blueberries, lemon juice and dextrose powder into a medium saucepan.

Combine well and bring to the boil and then simmer for approx. 15–20 minutes.

Allow to cool then transfer to a sterilised jar and seal.

Do not refrigerate as it will crystallise. Instead, store in cupboard.

Raspberry jam

Makes 1 jar

2 punnets raspberries

2 tbsp lemon juice

1¾ cups dextrose powder

Place the raspberries, lemon juice and dextrose powder into a medium saucepan and combine well.

Bring the mixture to the boil and then simmer for approx. 20–25 minutes.

Allow to cool then transfer to a sterilised jar and seal.

Do not refrigerate as it will crystallise. Instead, store in a cupboard.

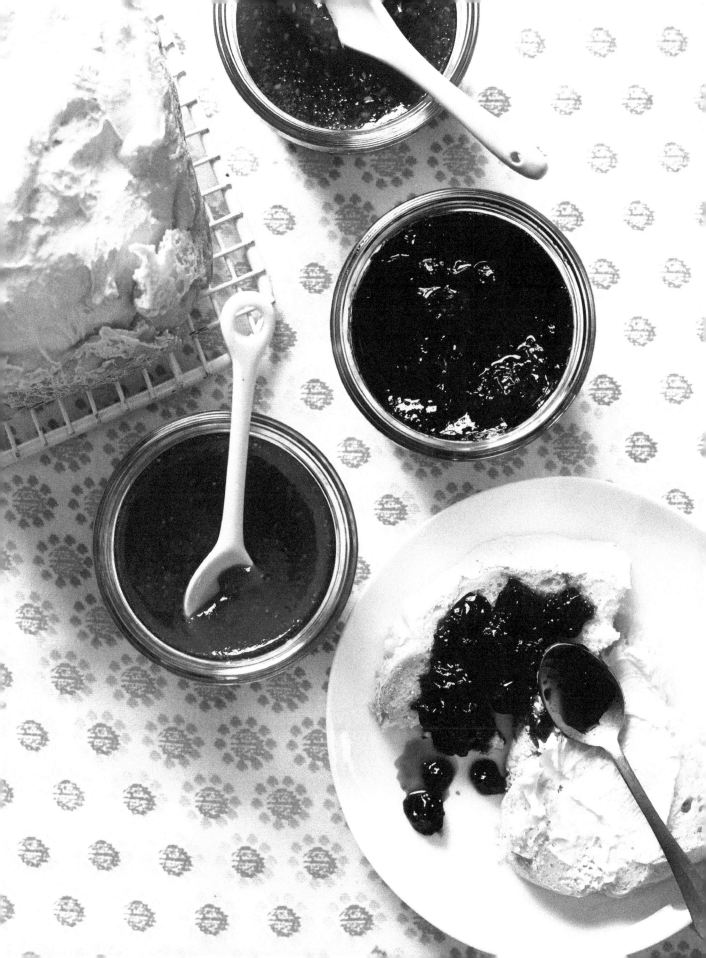

Strawberry jam

Makes 1 jar

2 punnets strawberries, hulled

2 cups dextrose powder

2 tbsp lemon juice

Place the hulled strawberries, lemon juice and dextrose powder in a blender and blend until it's a smooth consistency.

Pour the strawberry mixture into a medium saucepan.

Bring the mixture to the boil and then simmer for approx. 30–35 minutes.

Allow to cool then transfer to a sterilised jar and seal.

Do not refrigerate as it will crystallise. Instead, store in a cupboard.

Caramel sauce

Serves 12

⅓ cup water

2 cups dextrose powder

300ml thickened
lactose-free cream

Place the water and dextrose powder in a medium saucepan over a medium heat. The mixture will begin to melt and come to a boil.

Allow to boil for approx. 10–15 minutes or until mixture just starts to turn a light golden colour. When this happens, take it off the heat and, using a whisk, mix through the cream.

When mixture is well combined, either serve or allow to cool. Be very careful as the mixture will be extremely hot.

Serve.

Chocolate sauce

Serves 4

50g butter

½ cup dextrose powder

3 tbsps pure cocoa powder

1 tbsp thickened lactose-free cream

Place the butter in a small saucepan over low heat.

Once butter is melted, add dextrose and cocoa powder and combine well.

Finally, add cream and stir over heat until well incorporated.

Serve.

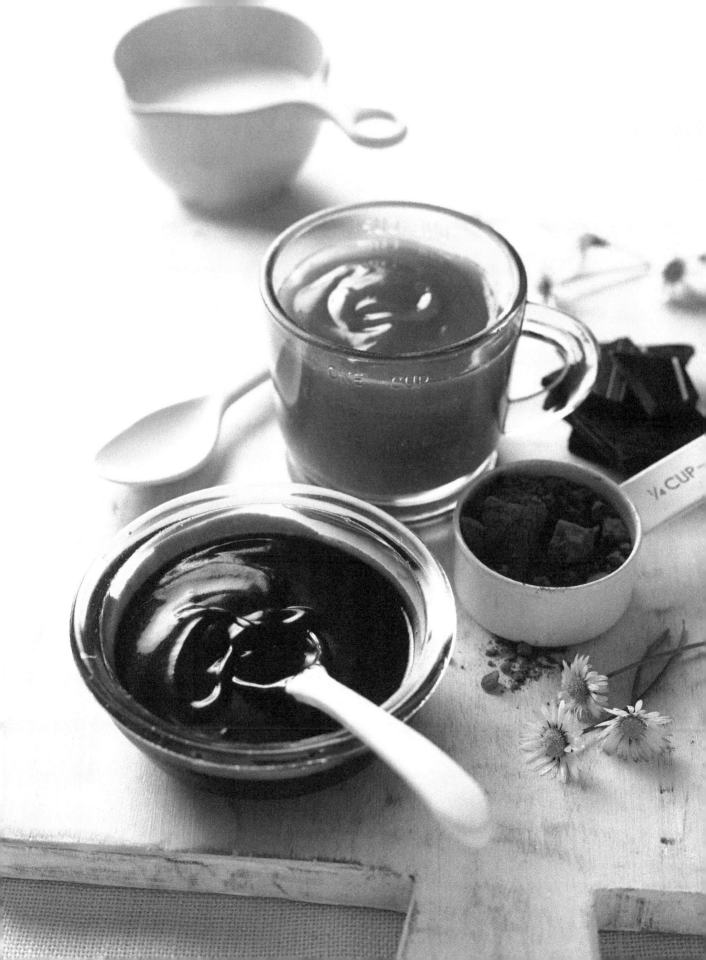

Chocolate brownies

Makes 12

175g butter, melted

¼ cup pure cocoa powder

1½ cups dextrose powder

3 eggs, beaten

½ tsp sugar-free pure vanilla extract

½ cup gluten-free plain flour

1 quantity chocolate sauce
(see recipe on page 108)

Preheat oven to 160°C.

Melt the butter in a medium saucepan, then add cocoa and dextrose powders. Combine well.

In a separate small bowl, mix the eggs and vanilla together.

Next, add flour into the butter mixture, and stir.

Finally, pour in egg mixture and incorporate well.

Pour mixture into a lined slice tin.

Cook for approx. 25–30 minutes.

Cool and top with chocolate sauce.

Serve.

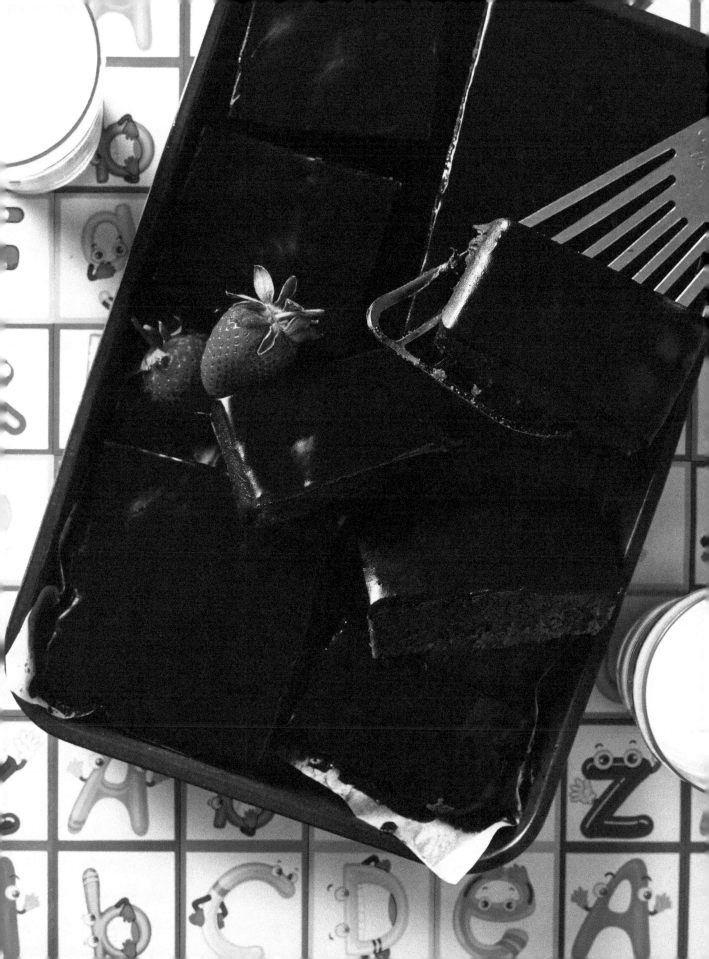

Chocolate cupcakes

Makes 12

2 cups gluten-free self-raising flour, sifted

1⅓ cups dextrose powder

¼ cup pure cocoa powder, sifted

½ tsp sugar-free pure vanilla extract

2 eggs

¾ cup lactose-free milk

125g butter, melted

Preheat oven to 180°C.

Place dry ingredients into a large mixing bowl and stir well.

In a separate small mixing bowl, combine the eggs, vanilla and milk.

Next, add the milk mixture to the dry ingredients and combine well.

Finally, pour in melted butter and ensure butter is completely incorporated.

Fill a patty pan-lined cupcake tray with tablespoons of the mixture.

Place in oven and cook for approx. 17–22 minutes or until a skewer inserted in the middle comes out clean.

Serve.

Vanilla cupcakes

Makes 12

2 cups gluten-free
self-raising flour, sifted

1⅓ cups dextrose powder

2 eggs, beaten

1 tsp sugar-free pure
vanilla extract

¾ cup lactose-free milk

125g butter, melted

Preheat oven to 180°C.

Combine the flour and dextrose powder in a large mixing bowl.

In a separate small mixing bowl, combine the eggs, vanilla and milk.

Pour egg mixture into the flour mixture and stir until well combined.

Next, stir in the melted butter until the mixture is smooth.

Place patty pans into a cupcake tin and spoon in the mixture.

Put the tray into the oven for approx. 17–22 minutes until cupcakes are golden brown on top.

Serve.

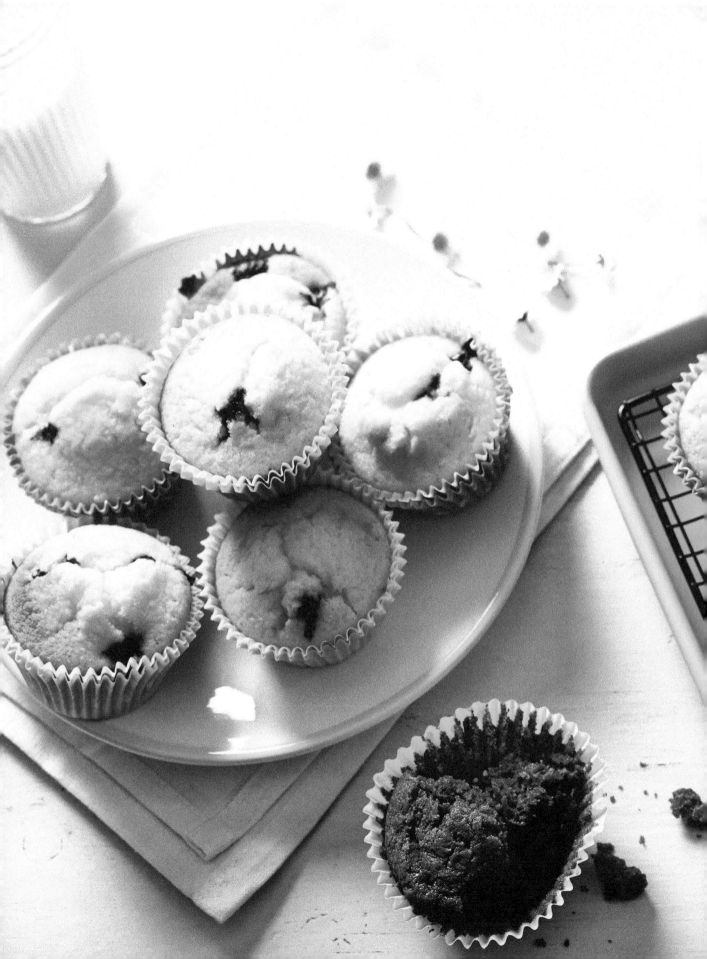

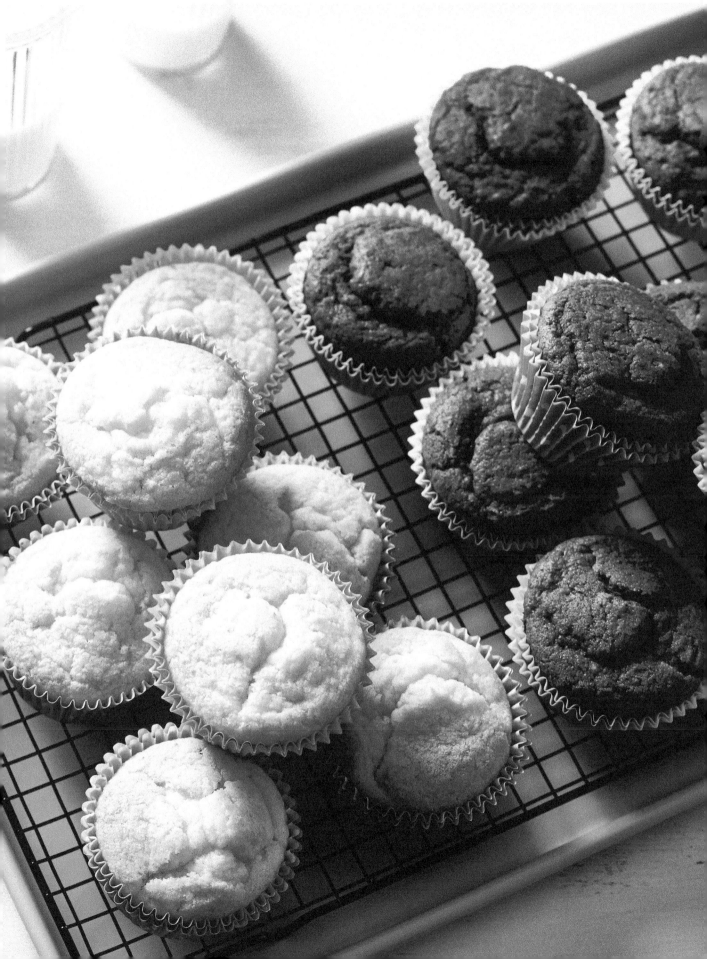

Vanilla and blueberry cupcakes

Makes 12

2 cups gluten-free
self-raising flour, sifted

1⅓ cups dextrose powder

2 eggs, beaten

1 tsp sugar-free pure
vanilla extract

¾ cup lactose-free milk

125g butter, melted

1 punnet blueberries

Preheat oven to 180°C.

Combine the flour and dextrose powder in a large mixing bowl.

In a separate small mixing bowl, combine the eggs, vanilla and milk.

Pour egg mixture into the flour mixture and stir until well combined.

Next, stir in the melted butter until the mixture is smooth. Then stir through the blueberries.

Place patty pans into a cupcake tin and spoon in the mixture.

Put the tray into the oven for approx. 20–25 minutes until cupcakes are golden brown on top.

Serve.

Banana ice-cream

Serves 10

1 cup lactose-free milk

1 cup dextrose powder

½ tbsp sugar-free pure vanilla extract

600ml thickened lactose-free cream

2½ bananas, medium, mashed (just ripened)

Into a mixer place milk, dextrose powder, vanilla, cream and banana. Mix on medium speed for approx. 1–2 minutes until really well combined.

Place in the fridge for at least 2 hours.

Put mixture into an ice-cream churner until it is ready.

Transfer to a container and freeze.

Chocolate ice-cream

Serves 10

1 cup lactose-free milk

1 cup dextrose powder

½ tbsp sugar-free pure vanilla extract

¼ cup pure cocoa powder

600ml thickened lactose-free cream

Into a mixer place milk, dextrose powder, vanilla, cocoa powder and cream. Mix on medium speed for approx. 1–2 minutes until really well combined.

Place in the fridge for at least 2 hours.

Put mixture into an ice-cream churner until it is ready.

Put in a container and freeze.

Serve.

Passionfruit ice-cream

Serves 10

1 cup lactose-free milk

1 cup dextrose powder

½ tbsp sugar-free pure vanilla extract

5 passionfruits, pulped

600ml thickened lactose-free cream

Into a mixer place milk, dextrose powder, vanilla, passionfruit and cream. Mix on medium speed for approx. 1–2 minutes until really well combined.

Place in the fridge for at least 2 hours.

Put mixture into an ice-cream churner until it is ready.

Put in container and freeze.

Serve.

Vanilla ice-cream

Serves 10

1 cup lactose-free milk

1 cup dextrose powder

1 tbsp sugar-free pure
vanilla extract

600ml thickened
lactose-free cream

Into a mixer place milk, dextrose powder, vanilla and cream. Mix on medium speed for approx. 1–2 minutes until really well combined.

Place in the fridge for at least 2 hours.

Put mixture into an ice-cream churner until it is ready.

Transfer to a container and freeze.

Serve.

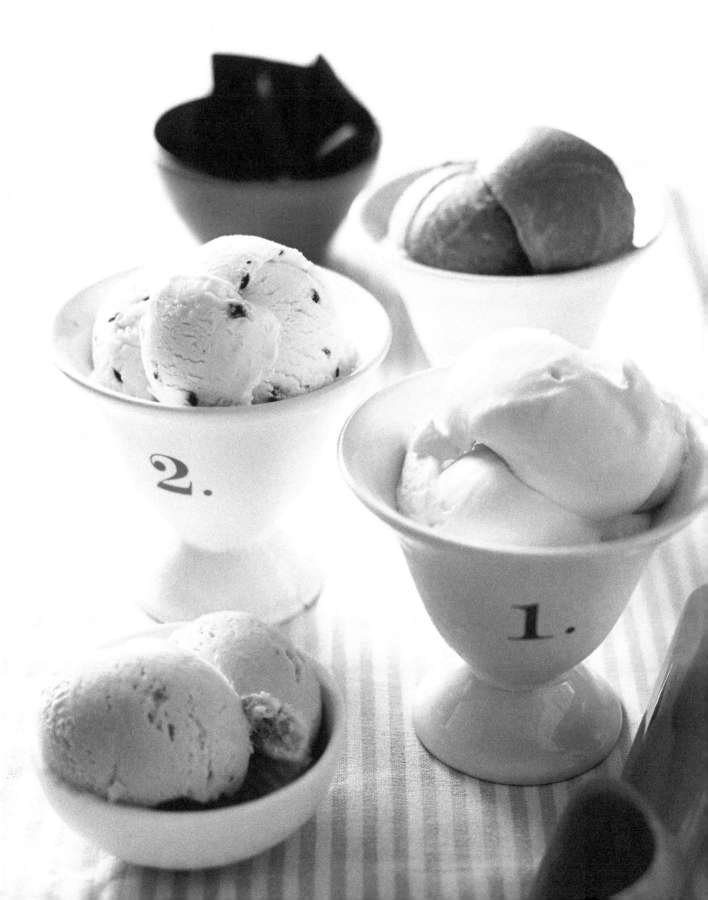

Fruit and marshmallow skewers

Makes 12

250g strawberries, sliced thickly

3 bananas, peeled and chopped into chunks (just ripened)

½ pineapple, peeled and chopped into chunks

4 kiwi fruits, peeled and chopped into chunks

1 quantity of marshmallows
(see recipe on page 128)

1 packet wooden skewers

Take the skewers and layer them with alternating pieces of fruit and marshmallow until ingredients are used up.

Serve.

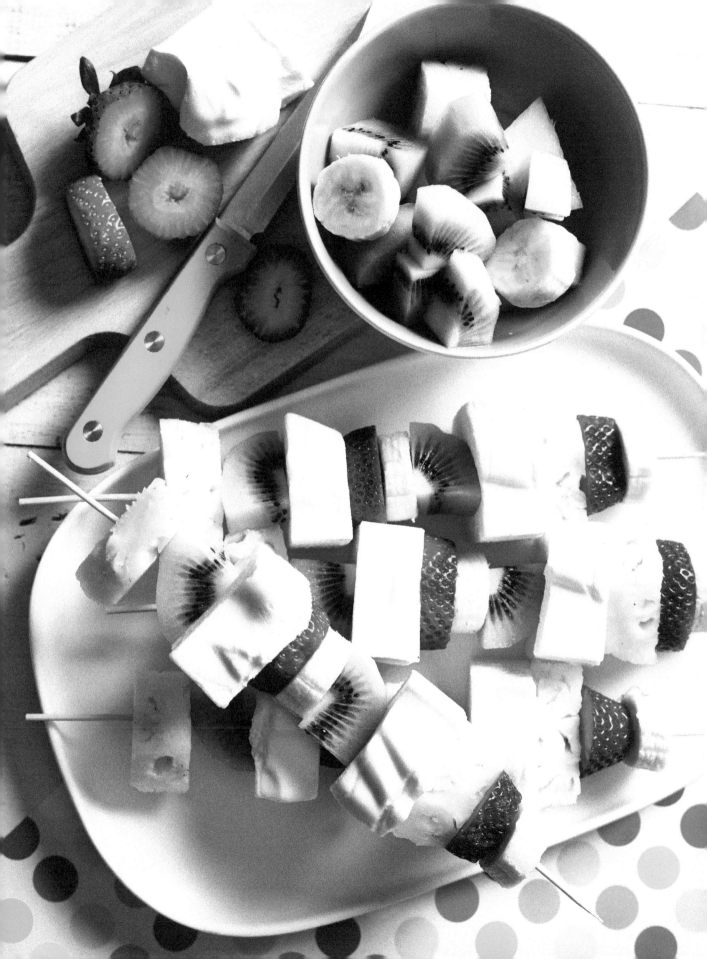

Chocolate mousse

Serves 8

600ml thickened
lactose-free cream

¼ cup pure cocoa powder,
sifted

1 cup dextrose powder

Pour the cream into a mixer and beat on medium speed until thickened.

Next, add the cocoa and dextrose powders and mix until well combined.

Place in refrigerator for at least 2 hours.

Serve.

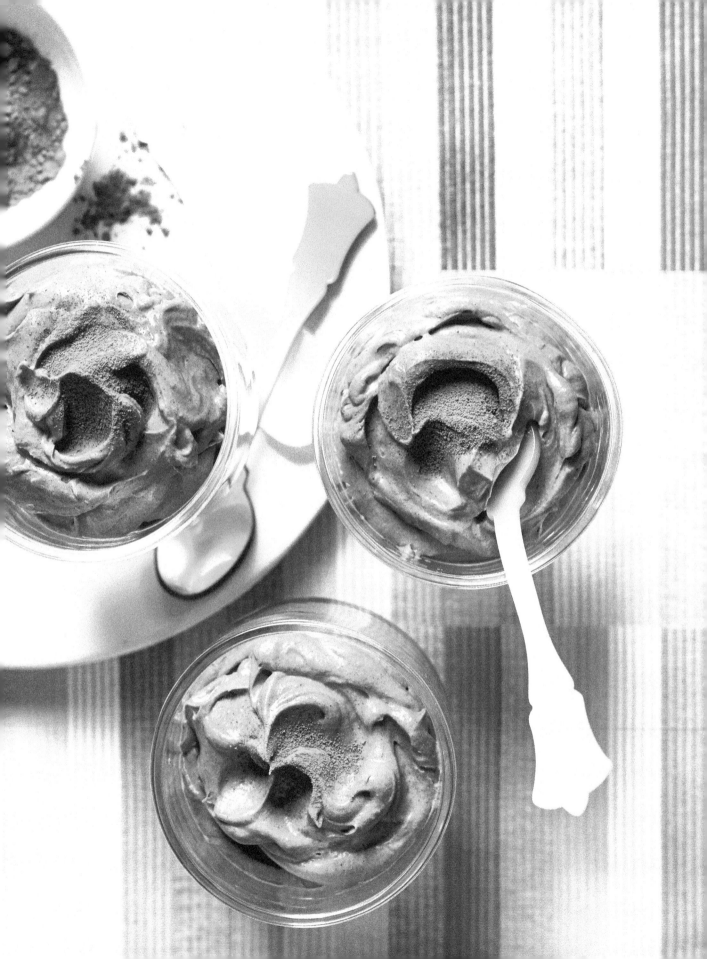

Lemon slice

Makes 16 slices

1 quantity vanilla biscuits
(see recipe on page 85),
crushed

**½ cup sweetened
condensed milk**
(see recipe on page 152)

2 lemons, rind grated

2 cups dextrose powder

4 tbsp lemon juice

Into a large mixing bowl, place the vanilla biscuits, condensed milk and the grated rind of 1 lemon. Incorporate well.

Place biscuit mixture into a lined slice tin, squashing in firmly, and place in the fridge.

Next, into a small saucepan add the dextrose powder, lemon juice and the rind of the remaining lemon.

Over a low heat, combine well until the mixture is just beginning to melt but still white in colour. Pour over the biscuit base and place back in fridge for approx. 1 hour or until well set.

Slice and serve.

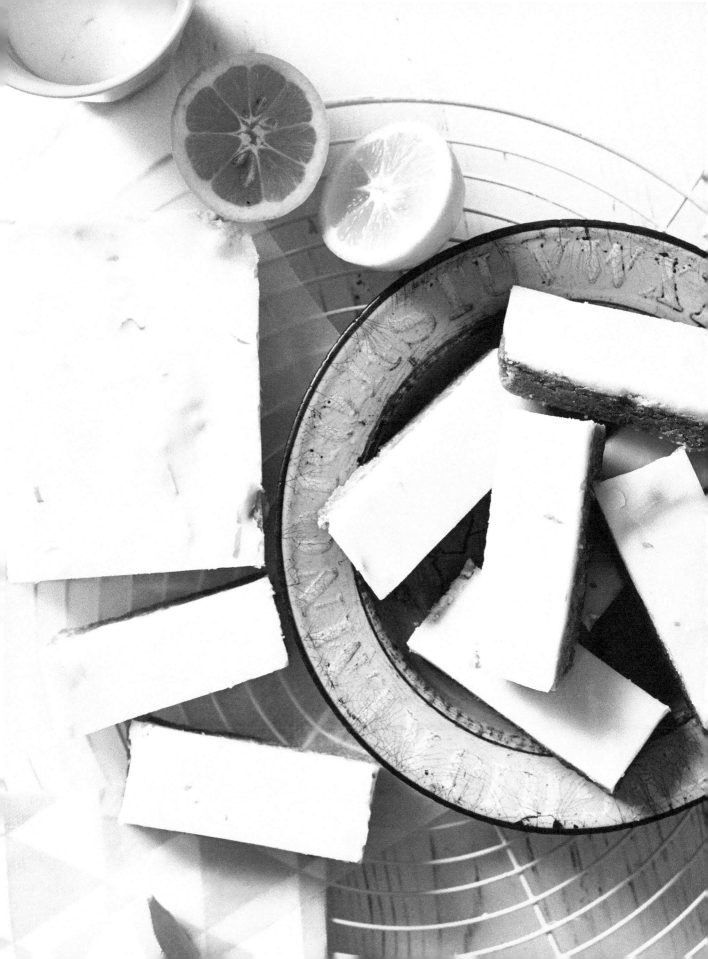

Marshmallows

Makes 20 pieces

160ml water

2 cups dextrose powder

⅓ cup hot water

20g powdered gelatin

2 large eggs
(use egg whites only)

1 tsp sugar-free vanilla
extract

Pour 160ml water and the dextrose powder into a medium saucepan over a medium heat and allow dextrose to dissolve.

Bring mixture to boil without stirring, but watch it until the mixture reaches 120°C on a sugar thermometer.

While the sugar mixture is boiling, put the ⅓ cup of hot water into a mixing bowl. Gradually whisk the gelatin into the hot water until dissolved.

In an electric mixer, beat egg whites until soft peaks form.

When sugar mixture has reached 120°C, remove from heat. Whisk in the gelatin mixture until well combined. Pour this combined mixture into a heatproof pouring jug.

On a low speed, gradually pour the dextrose mixture into the beaten egg whites. Turn mixer onto high speed and continue mixing for 10 minutes, until the mixture is thick and cool. Add vanilla essence to mixture and stir until combined.

Line a slice tin with baking paper then pour in the mixture and smooth with a spatula.

Refrigerate for 5 hours. Slice and serve.

Peanut brittle

Makes 16 pieces

2 cups dextrose powder

50g butter, diced

150g peanuts, unsalted

Place dextrose powder into a medium saucepan, melt and bring to the boil for 10–12 minutes until the mixture starts to turn a golden colour and temperature reaches 150°C.

Take the mixture off the stove and whisk through the butter.

Next, incorporate the peanuts and pour into a lined slice tin.

Place in the refrigerator until hard.

Break into pieces and serve.

Toffees

Makes 12

⅓ cup water

2 cups dextrose powder

½ tbsp lemon juice

Place water, dextrose powder and lemon juice into a medium saucepan.

Bring the mixture to a boil then turn down to a simmer. Simmer until the mixture begins to turn golden brown and temperature reaches 150°C, approx. 10 minutes.

Place mini patty pans into a mini cupcake tin and grease to stop from sticking. Pour mixture into patty pans and place in refrigerator for at least 3 hours.

Serve.

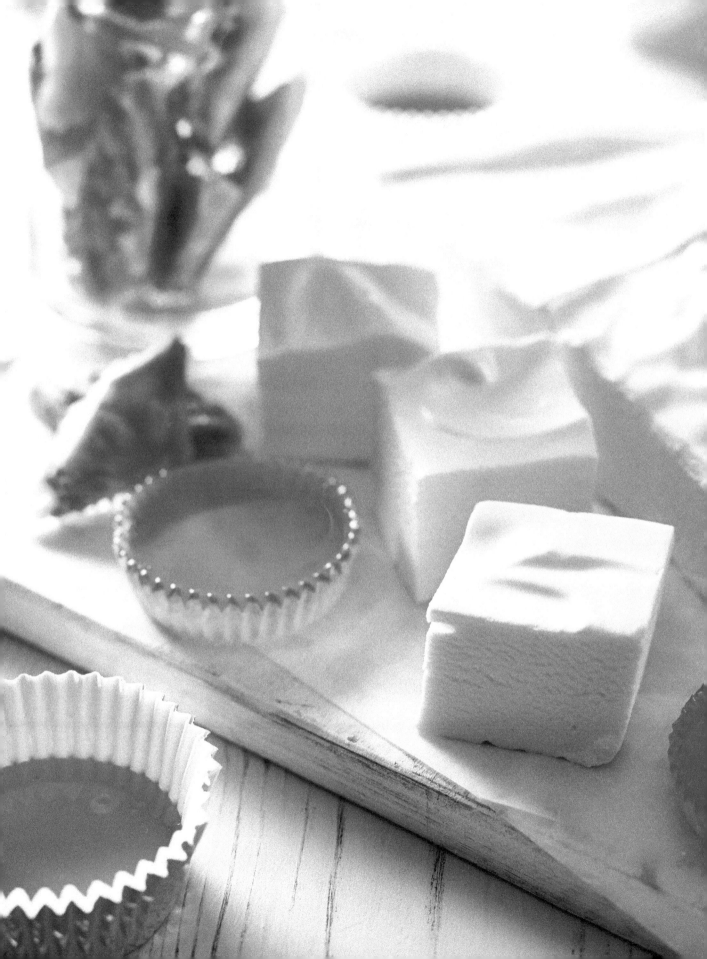

Mixed berry and banana sorbet

Serves 4

1½ bananas, peeled and sliced (just ripened)

125g blueberries

250g strawberries, halved

Place banana, blueberries and strawberries in a container with a lid and put into the freezer overnight or until frozen.

Place frozen fruit into a blender and blend well, ensuring to scrape down the sides at regular intervals.

Once the mixture is a smooth consistency and has come together to a sorbet consistency, the sorbet is ready.

Serve.

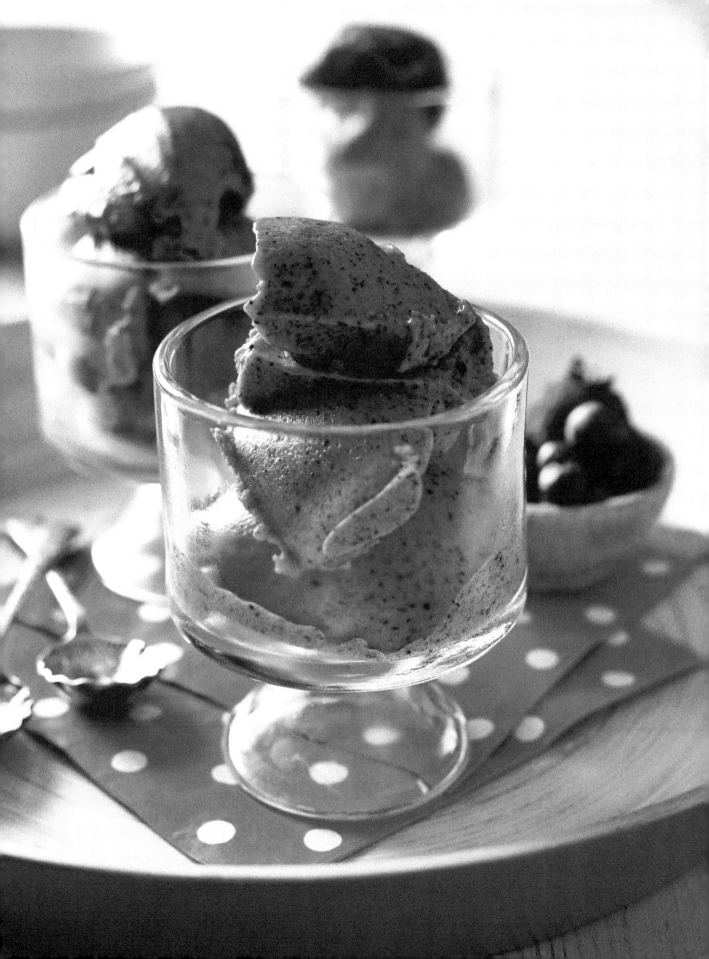

Blueberry cheesecake

Serves 10

½ **batch of
shortbread biscuits**
(see recipe on page 84)

40g butter, melted

**1 punnet blueberries,
hulled**

1 cup dextrose powder

**375g lactose-free cream
cheese**

2¾ tsp powdered gelatin

2 tbsp boiled water

Process biscuits in a food processor until fine crumbs.

Add melted butter and mix well.

Line a 19cm springform tin with baking paper at the base.

Pour crumb mixture into tin and pack firmly. Place in refrigerator for 5 minutes.

Next, place blueberries and dextrose powder in a blender and combine until smooth.

Add cream cheese, blend until smooth.

In a small bowl place gelatin and boiled water and stir until combined.

Pour the gelatin mixture into blueberry mixture and blend.

Finally, pour blueberry mixture over biscuit crumb base.

Place in refrigerator overnight to set.

Serve.

Raspberry cheesecake

Serves 10

½ **batch of**
shortbread biscuits
(see recipe on page 84)

40g butter, melted

1 punnet raspberries

1 cup dextrose powder

375g lactose-free cream
cheese

2¾ tsp powdered gelatin

2 tbsp boiled water

Process biscuits in a food processor until fine crumbs. Add melted butter and mix well.

Line a 19cm springform tin with baking paper at the base. Pour crumb mixture into tin and pack firmly. Place in refrigerator for 5 minutes.

Next, place the raspberries and dextrose powder in a blender and process until smooth. Add the cream cheese and again blend until smooth.

Place the gelatin and boiled water in a small mixing bowl and stir until combined.

Pour the gelatin mixture into the raspberry mixture and blend.

Finally, pour the raspberry mixture over the biscuit crumb base.

Place in refrigerator overnight to set.

Serve.

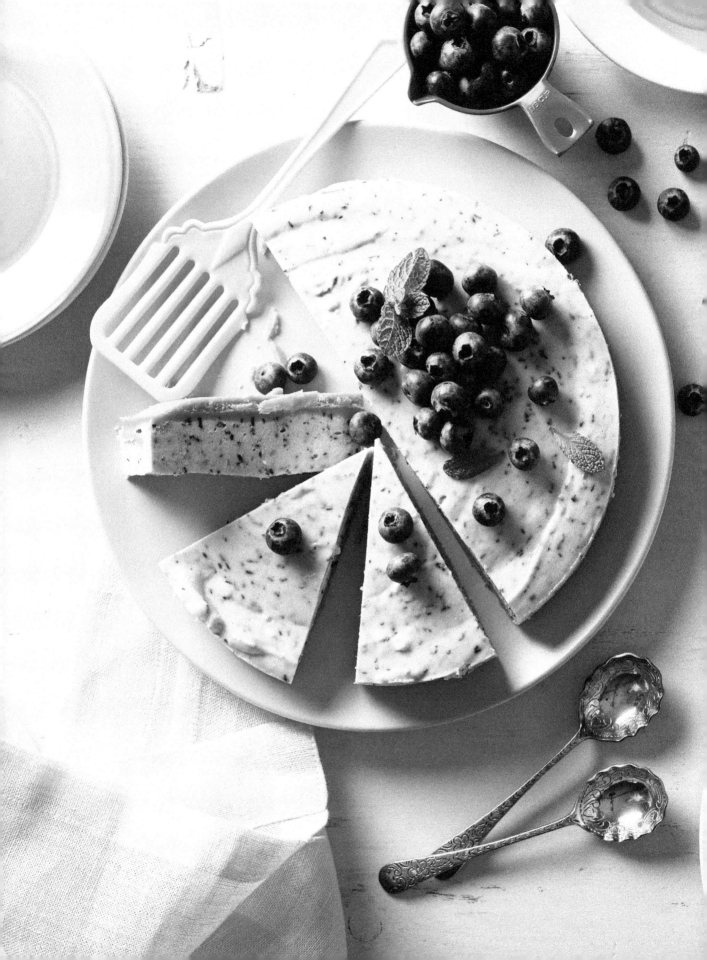

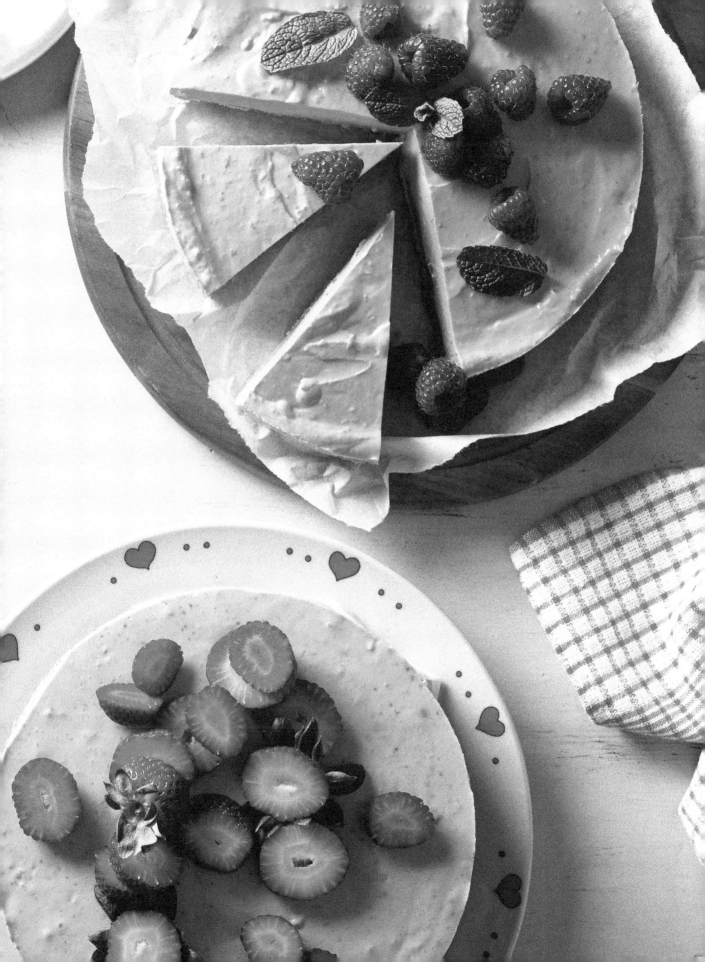

Strawberry cheesecake

Serves 10

½ **batch of
shortbread biscuits**
(see recipe on page 84)

40g butter, melted

**1 punnet strawberries,
hulled**

1 cup dextrose powder

**375g lactose-free cream
cheese**

2¾ tsp powdered gelatin

2 tbsp boiled water

Process biscuits in a food processor until fine crumbs.
Add melted butter and mix well.

Line a 19cm springform tin with baking paper at the base.
Pour crumb mixture into tin and pack firmly. Place in
refrigerator for 5 minutes.

Next, place the strawberries and dextrose powder in a
blender and process until smooth. Add the cream cheese
and again blend until smooth.

Place the gelatin and boiled water in a small mixing bowl
and stir until combined.

Pour the gelatin mixture into the strawberry mixture
and blend.

Finally, pour the strawberry mixture over the biscuit
crumb base.

Place in refrigerator overnight to set.

Serve.

Orange fizzy drink

Serves 2

1 orange, juiced

2 tbsp dextrose powder

250ml carbonated water

Place orange juice, dextrose powder and carbonated water into a jug. Stir until well combined.

Serve.

Orange and lemon fizzy drink

Serves 2

1 orange, juiced

½ lemon, juiced

2½ tbsp dextrose powder

250ml carbonated water

Place orange juice, lemon juice, dextrose powder and carbonated water into a jug. Stir until well combined.

Serve.

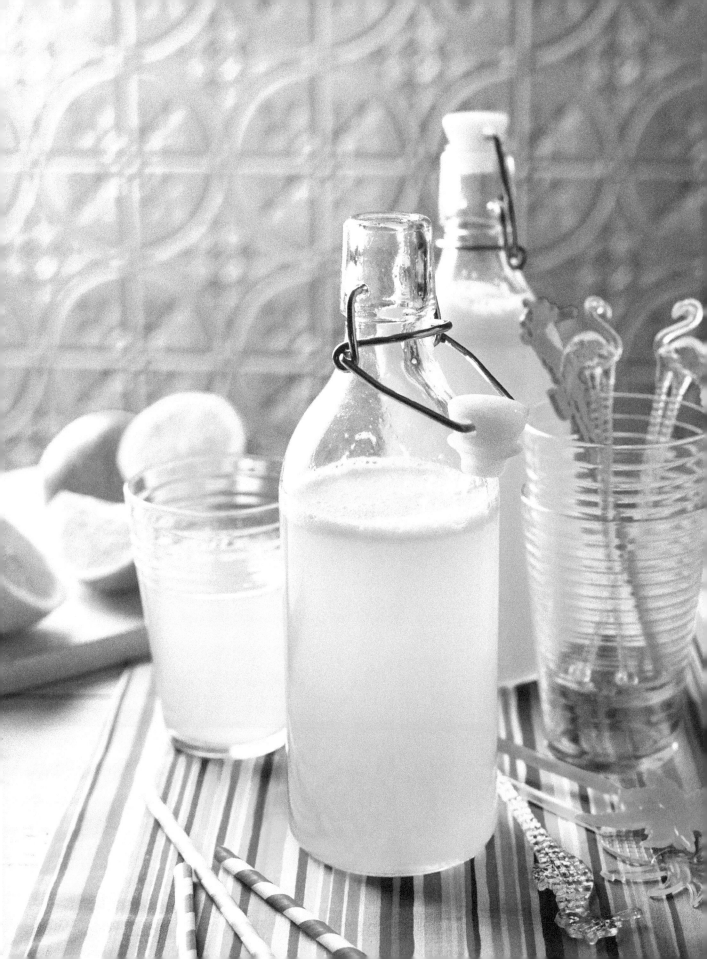

Pancakes

Makes 8

2 cups gluten-free
self-raising flour, sifted

1¾ cups lactose-free milk

1 cup dextrose powder

2 eggs

Butter

Combine flour, milk, dextrose powder and eggs in a large mixing bowl.

On a medium heat, place approx. 1 tsp of butter in a large frying pan and allow to melt and coat the base of the pan.

Pour a small amount of mixture into the pan, swirl around to spread evenly, and allow to cook.

When air bubbles begin to form on the surface of the pancake, use a spatula to flip the pancake over to cook the other side.

When both sides are golden brown, place on a plate and repeat with the remaining mixture.

Serve with pure maple syrup.

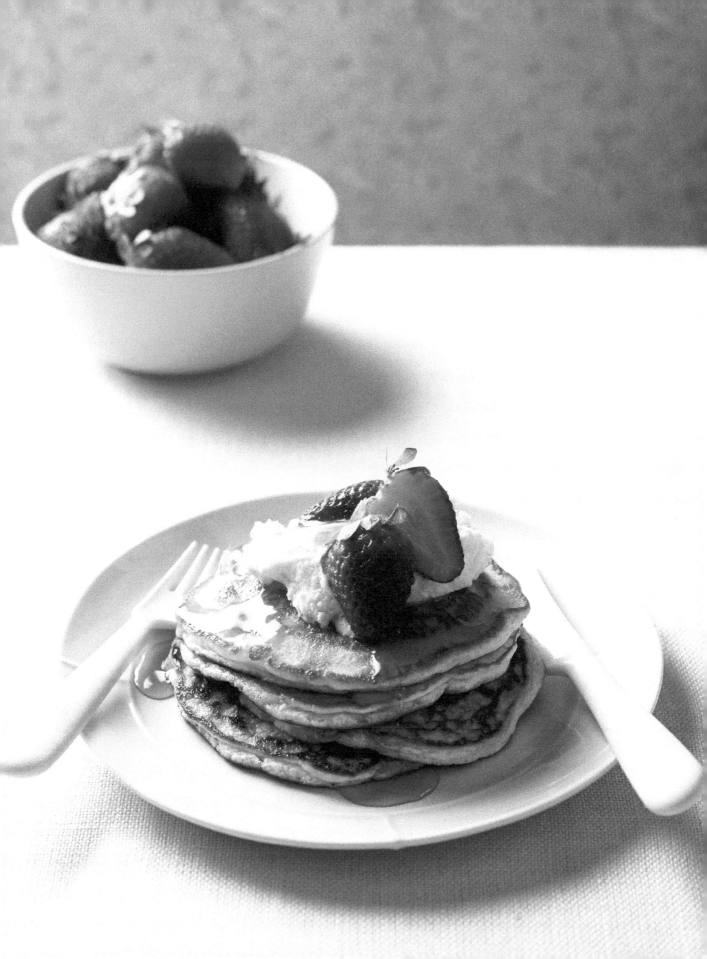

Pavlova with passionfruit cream

Serves 10

4 eggs, whites only

1¾ cups dextrose powder

1 tsp lemon juice

2 tsp gluten-free cornflour

600ml thickened lactose-free cream

½ tsp sugar-free pure vanilla extract

5 passionfruits, pulped

½ punnet strawberries, halved

½ punnet blueberries

Preheat oven to 110°C

Beat egg whites in a large mixing bowl for approx. 8 minutes until they are soft white peaks.

Slowly, 1 teaspoon at a time, incorporate 1½ cups of dextrose powder.

Next, add the cornflour and combine, and then add the lemon juice.

Spoon the mixture onto a lined baking tray and sculpt into the desired shape.

Place in oven for approx. 1 hour and 45 minutes then turn off oven and leave overnight.

Now, in a separate bowl, whisk the cream until thickened. Add remaining dextrose, vanilla extract and passionfruit pulp and whip until thick.

Spread cream mixture over the top of the pavlova and then top with blueberries and strawberries.

Serve.

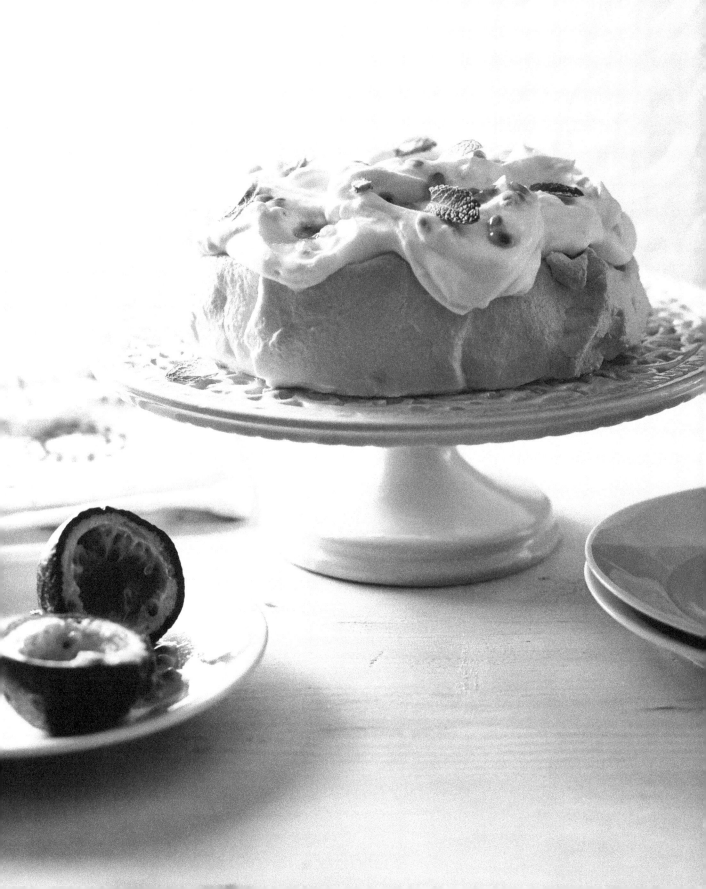

Rumballs

Makes 12

1 quantity vanilla biscuits
(see recipe on page 85)
crushed

2 tbsp pure cocoa powder

**½ cup sweetened
condensed milk**
(see recipe on page 152)

¼ cup shredded coconut

Into a large mixing bowl, place the biscuits, cocoa powder and condensed milk and combine well.

Roll the mixture into small balls.

Place the balls into a small mixing bowl with the coconut and coat.

Refrigerate for at least 1 hour, then serve.

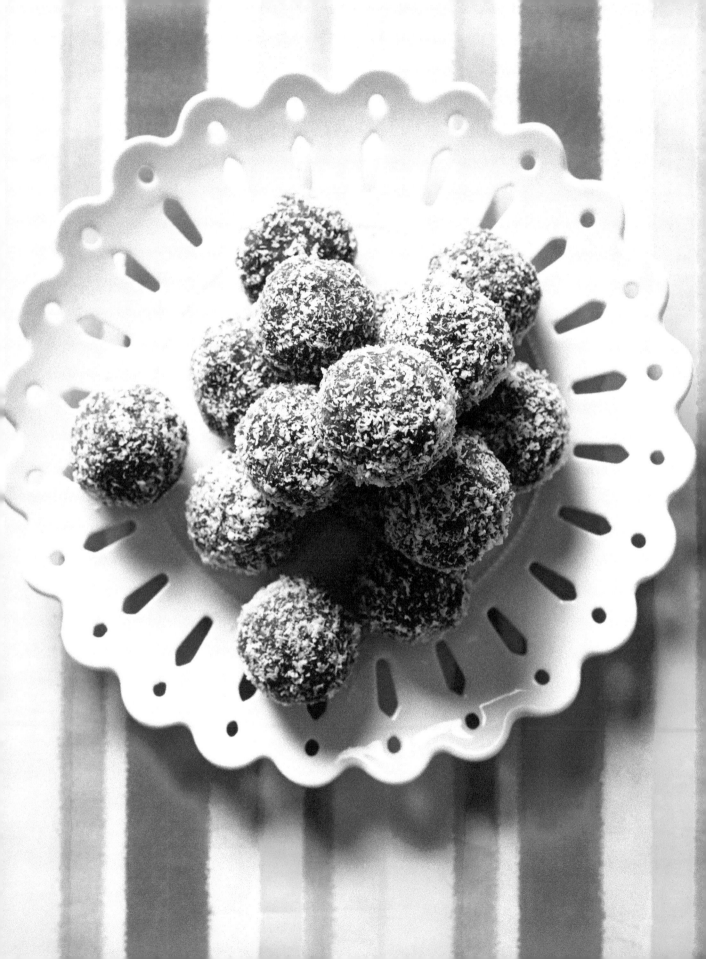

Scones with strawberry jam and cream

Makes 6

2 cups gluten-free self-raising flour

60g butter

¼ tsp salt

¾ cup lactose-free milk

Extra gluten-free flour for dusting

Strawberry jam
(see recipe on page 106)

Whipped cream
(see recipe on page 153)

Preheat oven to 180°C.

Into a mixer, place the flour, butter and salt, and combine well.

Pour in the milk and mix until incorporated.

On a bench, sprinkle some flour then turn out the mixture. Knead it down using extra flour if required until the dough is well formed. Roll out to approx. 4cm thickness and cut with a round cutter.

Place scones on a lined baking tray and put in the oven for approx. 25–30 minutes or until golden brown.

Cool and top with jam and cream.

Serve.

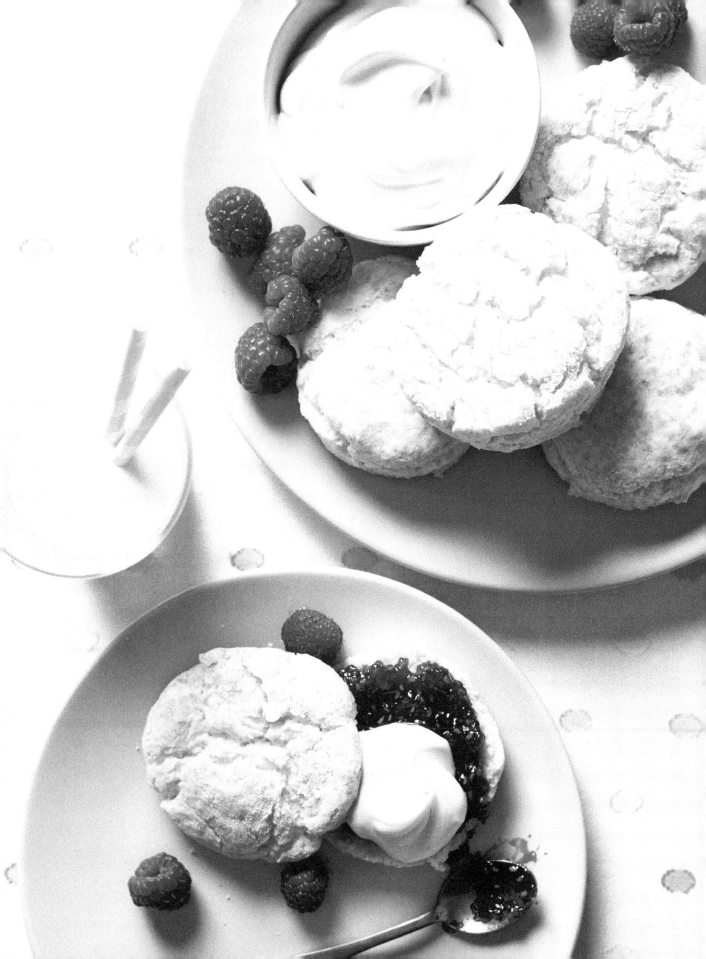

Vanilla and chocolate marble cake

Serves 10

2 cups gluten-free self-raising flour, sifted

1½ cups dextrose powder

2 eggs, beaten

1 tsp sugar-free pure vanilla extract

¾ cup lactose-free milk

125g butter, melted

2 tbsp pure cocoa powder

Chocolate icing

50g butter

½ cup dextrose powder

3 tbsps pure cocoa powder

1 tbsp thickened lactose-free cream

Preheat oven to 180°C.

Combine the flour and dextrose powder in a large mixing bowl.

In a separate small mixing bowl, combine the eggs, vanilla and milk.

Pour egg mixture into the flour mixture and stir until well combined.

Next, stir in the melted butter until the mixture is smooth.

Pour half of the mixture into a 19cm cake tin, then combine the cocoa powder with the remaining half.

Pour the chocolate mixture into the cake tin and, using a skewer, swirl it about to get a marbled texture.

Put the cake tin into the oven for approx. 45–50 minutes or until cake is golden brown on top and a skewer comes out clean when inserted in the middle.

Set aside to cool.

For the icing, place the butter in a small saucepan over a low heat.

Once butter has melted, add the dextrose and cocoa powders and combine well.

Finally, add the cream and stir over heat until well incorporated.

Wait 10 minutes then pour the icing over the cake.

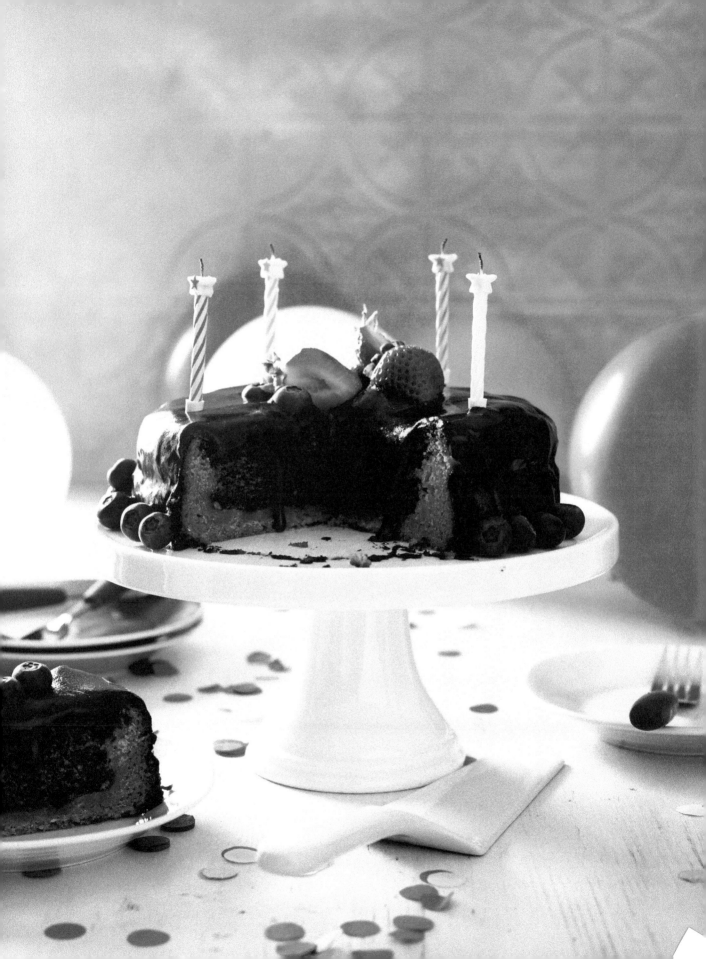

Sweetened condensed milk

Makes 3 cups

2 cups thickened lactose-free cream

50g butter

2½ cups dextrose powder

Over a medium heat, combine the cream, butter and dextrose powder in a medium saucepan. When ingredients are well combined, bring to the boil then turn to a low heat and allow to simmer for 25–30 minutes, stirring occasionally.

When ready, pour ingredients through a sieve and set aside to cool. This needs to be prepared and used on the same day.

Whipped cream

Serves 6

600ml thickened lactose-free cream

3 tbsp rice malt syrup

Place cream into a mixer and mix on medium speed until the cream has thickened. Next, add rice malt syrup and combine well. Serve.

Cook's notes

tsp	teaspoon (5ml)	biscuit tray	36 × 27cm
tbsp	tablespoon (15ml)	small mixing bowl	1.2 litre
cup	250ml	medium mixing bowl	2.8 litre
small pot	1.5 litre	large mixing bowl	3.5 litre
medium pot	2.5 litre	frying pan	26 cm
large pot	3.5 litre	stockpot	7.6 litre
slice tin	31 × 20cm	baking dish	4 litre

Festive meal plan

Pumpkin soup
Roast lamb veggies and gravy
Crusty crumbed chicken
Peri peri chicken
Cucumber and tomato salad
Strawberry cheesecake
Chocolate mousse
Blueberry crumble and custard
Baked custard
Pavlova and passionfruit cream
Orange fizzy drink
Orange and lemon fizzy drink
Vanilla ice-cream
Shortbread biscuits

Party meal plan

Tacos
Meatballs and salsa
Rice paper rolls
Mini pizzas
Tomato, cheese and chive muffins
Orange fizzy drink
Orange and lemon fizzy drink
Chocolate mousse
Chocolate cupcakes
Chocolate brownies
Lemon slice
Rumballs
Fruit and marshmallow skewers
Marshmallow
Toffee
Peanut brittle
Vanilla and chocolate marble cake with chocolate topping

Index

Banana
    Banana and blueberry cake 88
    Ice-cream 117
    Milkshake 90
    Mixed berry and banana sorbet 132
    Split 98
Beef
    Homemade hamburgers 36
    Lasagne 40
    Meat sauce and rice 70
    Meatballs and salsa dip 66
    Oven spaghetti 46
    Savoury rice 60
    Spaghetti Bolognese 62
    Stock 18
    Tacos 24
Biscuits
    Anzac 80
    Chocolate 81
    Gingernut 82
    Shortbread 84
    Vanilla 85
Blueberry
    Banana and blueberry cake 88
    Cheesecake 134
    Crumble 100
    Jam 103
Cake
    Banana and blueberry cake 88
    Pavlova with passionfruit cream 144
    Vanilla and chocolate marble cake 150
    See also Cheesecake, Cupcakes
Capsicums, stuffed 64
Caramel
    Milkshake 91
    Sauce 107
    Sundae 96
Cheesecake
    Blueberry 134
    Raspberry 135
    Strawberry 138
Chicken
    Chicken soup 28
    Chicken noodle soup 26
    Crusty crumbed chicken legs 22
    Peri peri chicken 48
    Red chicken 52
    Stock 20
Chocolate
    Biscuits 81
    Brownies 110
    Cupcakes 112
    Milkshake 92
    Mousse 124
    Sauce 108
    Sundae 97
    Vanilla and chocolate marble cake 150
Condensed milk, sweetened 152
Cottage pie 30
Cream, whipped 153
Crumble, blueberry 100

Cucumber
    Cucumber and cherry tomato salad 21
Cupcakes
    Chocolate 112
    Vanilla 113
    Vanilla and blueberry 116
Custard 102
    Baked custard 86
Drinks
    Milkshakes (*see* Milkshakes)
    Orange fizzy drink 139
    Orange and lemon fizzy drink 140
Eggs
    Egg and chive pasta with lamb
        cutlets 32
Hamburgers 36
Ice-cream
    Banana 117
    Chocolate 118
    Passionfruit 119
    Vanilla 120
Jam
    Blueberry 103
    Raspberry 104
    Strawberry 106
Lamb
    Cottage pie 30
    Egg and chive pasta with lamb
        cutlets 32
    Lamb stew 38
    Moussaka 44
    Roast lamb, veggies and gravy 58
Lasagne 40
Lemon slice 126
Marshmallow 128
    Fruit and marshmallow skewers 122
Milkshakes
    Banana 90
    Caramel 91
    Chocolate 92
    Strawberry 93
Moussaka 44
Mousse
    Chocolate 124
Muffins
    Tomato, cheese and chive 72
Pancakes 142
Passionfruit
    Ice-cream 119
    Pavlova with passionfruit cream 144
Pasta
    Egg and chive pasta with lamb
        cutlets 32
    Fettucine carbonara 34
    Lasagne 40
    Oven spaghetti 46
    Red spaghetti and meatballs 54
    Spaghetti Bolognese 62
Pavlova with passionfruit cream 144
Peanut brittle 129
Pizza, mini 42

Pumpkin
    Pumpkin soup 50
Raspberry
    Cheesecake 135
    Jam 104
Rice
    Rice paper rolls 56
    Savoury rice 60
Rumballs 146
Salad
    Cucumber and cherry tomato 21
    Tuna 76
Salsa, tomato 67
Sauce
    Bolognese 62
    Caramel 107
    Chocolate 108
Savoury rice 60
Scones with strawberry jam and cream
    148
Sorbet, mixed berry and banana 132
Soup
    Chicken 28
    Chicken noodle 26
    Pumpkin 50
Spaghetti
    Oven spaghetti 46
    Red spaghetti and meatballs 54
    Spaghetti Bolognese 62
Stew
    Lamb stew 38
Stock
    Beef 18
    Chicken 20
Strawberry
    Cheesecake 138
    Jam 106
    Milkshake 93
    Scones with strawberry jam
        and cream 148
Sundae
    Caramel 96
    Chocolate 97
Toffee 130
Tomato
    Bolognese Sauce 62
    Cucumber and cherry tomato salad 21
    Mini pizza 42
    Salsa 67
    Tomato, cheese and chive muffins 72
Tuna
    Tuna mornay 74
    Tuna salad 76
Vanilla
    Biscuits 85
    Vanilla and chocolate marble cake 150
    Cupcakes 113
    Vanilla and blueberry cupcakes 116

Acknowledgements

To Keira and Madison, you are the magnum opus of my life. I love you infinitely. I know things have been difficult but you have both been so amazing and strong, I am so proud to be your mum. This book is for you both.

To my husband William, I adore you. You are the love of my life. Thank you for always pushing me to do better and for believing in me even when I don't believe in myself. You are my rock and best friend.

To my parents, thank you for all that you do for me and my family. I can't tell you how comforting it is to know that you always have my back. I love you both. Mum, I couldn't have done this without you.

To my siblings, especially my sister Terran and cousin Nicolle, thank you for being so supportive; the listening ear and shoulder to cry on. To Virginia, thank you for your help with the book. To Prue, well you know why.

To all my taste testers, there were some hits and some misses but I hope you all had fun anyway.

To my fabulous paediatric dietitian Miriam Raleigh, you have literally been a life saver, you helped to simplify everything.

To Yalamber Limbu, you are a fantastic doctor and your support and discussions were invaluable. We need more doctors like you.

To Julie, Cherise, Michael and the team, the book looks amazing – thank you for all your hard work.

Finally, to Janelle Couch, Accredited Practising Dietitian. Thank you for your promptness and diligence in helping to make this book a reality. This wouldn't have been possible without you.

CPSIA information can be obtained
at www.ICGtesting.com
Printed in the USA
LVHW070520201220
674643LV00008B/361

9 780648 402480